Genders and Sexualities in History

Palgrave Macmillan's series, Genders and Sexualities in History, accommodates and fosters new approaches to historical research in the fields of genders and sexualities. The series promotes world-class scholarship, which concentrates upon the interconnected themes of genders, sexualities, religions/religiosity, civil society, politics and war.

Historical studies of gender and sexuality have, until recently, been more or less disconnected fields. In recent years, historical analyses of genders and sexualities have synthesised, creating new departures in historiography. The additional connectedness of genders and sexualities with questions of religion, religiosity, development of civil societies, politics and the contexts of war and conflict is reflective of the movements in scholarship away from narrow history of science and scientific thought, and history of legal processes approaches, that have dominated these paradigms until recently. The series brings together scholarship from Contemporary, Modern, Early Modern, Medieval, Classical and Non-Western History. The series provides a diachronic forum for scholarship that incorporates new approaches to genders and sexualities in history.

Rhian Elinor Keyse ·
Adeline Moussion Esteve · Emma Yapp
Editors

# Sexual Violence in Medicine and Psychiatry

## Addressing Harms Through Interdisciplinarity

palgrave
macmillan

*Editors*
Rhian Elinor Keyse
University of Wales Trinity Saint David
Carmarthen, UK

Adeline Moussion Esteve
Birkbeck, University of London
London, UK

Emma Yapp
University of Bristol
Bristol, UK

ISSN 2730-9479 ISSN 2730-9487 (electronic)
Genders and Sexualities in History
ISBN 978-3-032-10799-2 ISBN 978-3-032-10800-5 (eBook)
https://doi.org/10.1007/978-3-032-10800-5

This work was supported by Wellcome Trust.



This Palgrave Macmillan imprint is published by the registered company Springer Nature Switzerland AG
The registered company address is: Gewerbestrasse 11, 6330 Cham, Switzerland

# Series Editor Preface

In *Sexual Violence in Medicine and Psychiatry: Addressing Harms Through Interdisciplinarity*, editors Rhian Elinor Keyse, Adeline Moussion Esteve, Emma Yapp and the volume's contributors explore the ways medical, psychological, and psychiatric frames of meaning permeate modern understandings of sexual violence. In this interdisciplinary volume, the role of medical professionals and other regimes of power are analysed in local as well as global contexts, specifically the UK, US, Canada, Norway, Argentina, Kenya, Australia, and New Zealand. The authors are interested in the multiple ways medical and psychiatric knowledges have an impact on the treatment of people who have experienced sexual violence as well as on those who have perpetrated such harms. What is the role of medical professionals in criminal justice systems? How have the intersectional identities of victim-survivors and perpetrators influenced personal and institutional practices? The authors also explore how medical and psychiatric understandings of violence reproduce social dynamics of marginalisation. They situate shifts in the meaning of sexual violence within histories of feminism, colonialism, heteronormativity, and medical internationalism. Central to all the chapters are ways to resist systemic abuse and create more equitable, violence-free worlds.

An important addition to the "Gender and Sexualities in History" series, *Sexual Violence in Medicine and Psychiatry* contributes to our knowledge of the past in relation to questions about gender, medical authority, and sexual abuse.

# Acknowledgements

The editors wish to acknowledge the support of the Wellcome Trust [Grant number: 205378/Z/16/Z], which funded the Sexual Harms and Medical Encounters (SHaME) Project at Birkbeck, University of London, of which the editors were all part. We also thank the SHaME team for their support throughout this project: Joanna Bourke, Ruth Beecher, Rhea Sookdeosingh, Stephanie Wright, George Severs, Charlie Jeffries, and Allison McKibban.

# Contents

# Notes on Contributors

**Suzanne Egan** works in the School of Social Sciences, University of Western Sydney, Australia. Suzanne uses a post-structural theoretical and methodological approach to study the uptake of the trauma discourse in feminist work against sexual violence. The aim in undertaking this research programme is to bridge a gap between academic feminist scholarship and feminist work in applied settings.

**Lisa Featherstone** is a History Professor at the University of Queensland. She is working on sexuality, medicine and the law, and is currently researching sexual violence. Lisa co-leads the Australian Research Council Project "Responding to Sexual Harm: An Australian Historical Criminology Approach".

**Patsie Frawley** is an Associate Professor at the National Centre of Excellence in Intellectual Disability Health in the University of New South Wales. She is currently working on translating health information for people with intellectual disability, health professionals, and the community and undertaking research with women with disabilities on accessible violence response services, and reproductive coercive abuse.

**Heather R. Hlavka** is a Professor of Criminology and Law Studies in the Department of Social and Cultural Sciences at Marquette University. She researches sexual violence, trauma, law, science, and society, children and youth, feminist ethics, and transformative justice.

**Andy Kaladelfos** (They/Them) is a Senior Lecturer in Criminology in the School of Law, Society and Criminology, University of New South Wales, and Co-Convenor of the Gendered Violence Research Network. Andy co-leads the Australian Research Council Project "Responding to Sexual Harm: An Australian Historical Criminology Approach".

**Rhian Elinor Keyse** is a Lecturer in Global Historical Studies at the University of Wales Trinity St David. She is a social and cultural historian of gender in modern West and East Africa, and her current research focuses on histories of gender-based violence in Ghana and Kenya.

**Solveig Laugerud** is an Associate Professor in the Department of Criminology and Sociology of Law at the University of Oslo. Her research interests are knowledge production and use at the intersection of law, science, and technology in relation to institutional responses to crime victims.

**Adeline Moussion Esteve** is a Postdoctoral Researcher at Birkbeck, University of London. She works at the crossroads of critical trauma studies and research into sexual violence and domestic violence in the european context.

**Sameena Mulla** is an Associate Professor of Women's, Gender, and Sexuality Studies at Emory University. She examines gender, race, and power, and the intersections of law and health-care in U.S. interventions into sexual violence.

**Stéphanie Pache** is a Professor of Gender and Sexuality Studies at the Université du Québec à Montréal. After writing a history of feminist therapy, her current research examines the role of psy disciplines in feminist politics against gender violence.

**Gethin Rees** is a Senior Lecturer in sociology at Newcastle University. He is interested in the ways that medicine is employed in legal decision-making contexts, including the case of doctors and nurses conducting forensic investigation in sexual assault cases.

**George J. Severs** is a historian of sexual health, sexual violence and HIV/AIDS. He is a Postdoctoral Researcher at the Geneva Graduate Institute in Switzerland, where he is working on the history of race and sexual and reproductive health in postwar Britain. Before this, George worked at Birkbeck, University of London as a postdoctoral researcher on the

SHaME project. His first book *Radical Acts: HIV/AIDS Activism in Late Twentieth-Century Britain* was published in 2024.

**Joanna Zofia Spyra** is a PhD Candidate at the University of Bergen. Her dissertation investigates the interplay of health, sexuality, and Jewish philanthropy in 1930s Argentina.

**Deborah White** is a Sociology Professor at Trent University working at the intersection of science, medicine and law. Her research focuses on the institutional and technological responses to sexual violence, particularly medico-legal interventions.

**Natalie Wortley** specialises in the teaching and practice of criminal law, evidence and procedure. Formerly an Associate Professor at Northumbria University, she is now a District Tribunal Judge. She also sits as a Deputy District Judge in the magistrates' courts and is a lecturer for the Judicial College.

**Emma Yapp** is a Senior Research Associate at the University of Bristol. Their research interests include critical feminist theory, sexual violence, mental health, socio-legal scholarship, and critical disability theory. Their current research concerns trauma, sexual violence, justice, and power in the UK.

# List of Figures

## Challenging Ideas of 'Vulnerability' in Prevention of Violence Through the Stories, Experiences and Advocacy of Women with Disabilities

# Introduction

*Rhian Elinor Keyse, Adeline Moussion Esteve, and Emma Yapp*

## 1 Introduction[1]

Understandings of sexual violence, medicine, and psychiatry are increasingly entangled. Medical and psychiatric professionals, ideas, and interventions play a crucial role in responses to sexual violence: they are key in the care (or lack thereof) received by victims and survivors in the aftermath of assault; in forensic evidence gathering during investigations (Corrigan 2013; Mulla 2014); and in medical witness testimony in the criminal legal system (Hlavka and Mulla 2021). Medical and psychiatric

R. E. Keyse (✉)
University of Wales Trinity St David, Wales, UK
e-mail: r.keyse@uwtsd.ac.uk

A. Moussion Esteve
Birkbeck, University of London, London, UK
e-mail: a.moussion@bbk.ac.uk

E. Yapp
University of Bristol, Bristol, UK
e-mail: emma.yapp@bristol.ac.uk

[1] A statement is required clarifying that these editors are listed in alphabetical order, and all contributed equally to the volume.





R. E. Keyse et al. (eds.), *Sexual Violence in Medicine and Psychiatry*, Genders and Sexualities in History,
https://doi.org/10.1007/978-3-032-10800-5_1

discourses also inform wider societal discourses around sexual violence, evidenced by the increasing dominance of notions of psychological trauma in understandings of rape and sexual assault, and the primacy attached to forensic evidence of sexual violence. This collection explores how medical and psychiatric knowledge, practitioners, and practices engage with sexual violence and, more precisely, how the medical and psychiatric fields can reproduce social dynamics of marginalisation. The book thus expands analyses of sexual violence at the individual level of victims and perpetrators, to explore how medical and psychological ideas, and psychiatric models and institutions, also contribute to experiences of sexual violence and to the reproduction of socially harmful dynamics.

The contributors examine several core questions: how, when, and where, does sexual violence come to be within the remit of health professionals? What is the role of medical and psychiatric professionals within the criminal legal system? How have medical and psychiatric forms of knowledge influenced perceptions of sexual violence, the people who experience it, and the perpetrators of such violence? What have been the implications of medical and psychiatric approaches to sexual violence for people who have experienced such violence? How does attention to intersectionality impact our understanding of these implications (noting that the volume pays attention to issues of race, sexuality, mental health and illness, (dis)ability, gender, and class)? In responding to these questions, the contributors highlight the power dynamics inherent in medical and psychiatric "expertise", and how it is not just sexual violence in itself, but also the ways societies have responded to it even through seemingly care-oriented responses, which can be harmful.

Medical and psychiatric professionals take on an air of objectivity and self-evident truth, and are afforded the aura of expertise, even though there is little correlation between the presence of forensic evidence and the outcomes of sexual violence cases (Du Mont and Parnis 2000; Quinlan 2017; Mulla 2014). However, medicine and psychiatry are replete with relationships of domination (Hlavka and Mulla 2021; Nordstrom 1996). Medical knowledge around sexual violence has been (mis)used to produce typologies of "good" and "bad" victims based on compliance with medical interventions and evidence gathering (Mulla 2014; Sweet 2021); to call into question victims' and survivors' testimonies (Das 2003); and to reproduce and reinforce racialised and gendered hierarchies, which take on particular valences in colonial and postcolonial contexts (Pande 2012; Kolsky 2010; Singh 2021). When medical and psychiatric categories are perceived as objective facts, this obscures their instantiation within wider dynamics of power that determine *whose* experiences of sexual violence are taken seriously. The following chapters, in contrast, invite the reader to peel back this veneer of objectivity and speak to some of the ways in which medical and psychiatric knowledge has been used in normative, exclusionary, and harmful ways. Contributions shine a light on the specific ways particular discourses and interventions have emerged, thus demonstrating how "objective" and "scientific" medical responses to sexual violence are historically and contextually contingent.

We, as editors, see this collection as a call to recalibrate certain stories that feminism tells about sexual violence and medicine, and to scrutinise the stories that medicine and psychiatry tell about their past, as well as what the consequences of all these enmeshed and entangled narratives are for the lived experience of sexual violence. As a paradigmatic case, the story of the advent of the language of trauma, and how it lent impetus to Western feminist movements, highlights these entanglements; the subjects they speak of; and what they obscure. The story of the "discovery" of sexual trauma often starts with the consciousness-raising of the 1970s and 80s. It tells of the role that feminist psychiatrists such as Judith Herman played in formulating the diagnosis of post-traumatic stress disorder (PTSD), and later, the development of the special category of "complex" trauma, to emphasise both the unique harm caused by sexual violence, as well as the gendered nature of its occurrence (Herman 1992, 2015). Yet this story obscures the work of myriad women of colour that came before the 1970s, and the centrality of that work to knowledge production on sexual violence (Berenstain 2020; Phipps 2020). This story also hides the fact that the very definition of trauma is bound up with colonial, and heteronormative, logics (Goozee 2021; Sweet 2021). The very category of PTSD was produced by research dominated by white middle-class women (e.g. Burgess and Holmstrom 1974), and understandings of PTSD continue to reflect societal ideas about who the "normal" victim of sexual violence is, namely: cis, white, middle-class, femme, sane, able… the list goes on (Spurgas 2021). The story of sexual trauma is just one of myriad stories that we tell about sexual violence, medicine, and psychiatry that have normative, and hence exclusionary, consequences (Butler 1992, 15–16). This collection of essays is a call to turn a critical eye towards both these stories, and medical and psychiatric categories and practices themselves.

Documenting dynamics of power in the forms of colonialism, white supremacy, and heteronormativity necessitates a transnational and interdisciplinary collection. The intersections between sexual violence and global health have been reinforced in international discussions around responses to the HIV/AIDS pandemic (UNAIDS 2022); access to healthcare for survivors of sexual violence in conflict and humanitarian crises (Marsh et al. 2006); and the global increase in sexual violence during the Covid-19 pandemic (UN Women 2020). This volume includes contributions covering Europe, North America, South America, Australasia, and Africa. Yet, this very book is also informed by the dynamics it examines. Several contributions originated from a symposium on sexual violence, medicine, and psychiatry held in 2020. The discussions on the day highlighted some of the nuanced ways in which the entanglements of these fields operate, and brought scholars together online from around the world. We, as editors, must draw the reader's attention to the fact that the majority of the chapters are written by academics working in the UK, Europe, North America, and Australia. This reflects more general biases within the literature on sexual violence, and academia in general (Demeter 2020). We made efforts to commission chapters from scholars working in the Global South, but as time went on, submissions were sparse, and we continued to receive more and more emails from scholars expressing their regret that they had to drop out. This in itself reflects issues of resources, how they contribute to what is known, and who gets to produce that knowledge (Medie and Kang 2018). We ask the reader to reflect on this as you engage with this collection, and acknowledge our position within this scholarly landscape.

As editors, we also want to acknowledge the broader context of violence, medicine, and psychiatry within which this work was created. The symposium which sparked these conversations took place during the Covid-19 pandemic, which revealed several forms of violence ranging from national policies to domestic violence, and a global increase in sexual violence (UN Women 2020). Since the pandemic, campaigns of disabling and debilitating violence have, and still are, occurring internationally. The questions of how "violence" is defined, responded to, and who gets to define it are still open. European colonisation has historically disrupted precolonial ways of knowing and defining violence: for example, settler colonial epistemologies exclude violence done to land, which is central to indigenous epistemologies, and as Nora Berenstain notes, this is "no accident" (Berenstain 2020, 735). We cannot have a conversation about sexual violence, colonialism, and the medical without acknowledging that these are live and continuing issues across the globe. The issues raised throughout this volume take on an urgency when considered in the context of contemporary violence: the ongoing genocide and colonial occupation of Palestine with the associated destruction of medical facilities and lack of reproductive justice for Palestinians (Office of the United Nations High Commissioner for Human Rights 2024); the violence in Sudan which has resulted in mass displacement, famine, and reports of widespread gender-based violence (Human Rights Watch 2024); sexual violence perpetrated as part of Russia's imperialist invasion of Ukraine (Busol 2023); rising incidences of violence against women and girls in the Democratic Republic of the Congo (Lederer 2024); and the forced sterilisation of Uyghur women in the Xinjiang region of China (Basu 2024). We also note with horror the ongoing impact of the repeal of *Roe v. Wade* for reproductive justice in the United States of America, and the particular repercussions for marginalised people and for victims and survivors of sexual violence (Lakshmi 2024). This is just a small number of cases, and the harms attached to such violence extend far beyond the medical and psychological.

## 2 Structure of the Book

The book is divided into three sections. The first section documents the diffusion and application of medical and psychiatric knowledge in prevention and intervention contexts, highlighting both its appeal and limitations. Non-medical professionals utilise psychological, psychiatric and medical knowledge on gender-based violence and sexual violence. Together, these chapters highlight the numerous ways in which psycho-medical knowledge is adopted and adapted by social actors, how this hybridisation complicates our understandings of both the harms of sexual violence and of the solutions to respond to it and invite us to rethink sexual violence beyond a psycho-medical gaze. Medical, psychological and psychiatric tools have been appropriated in many ways, and so this section leaves room for an exploration of the possibilities, and harms, of applications of this knowledge. The first two chapters explore the entanglements of psychology with feminism, blur the boundaries between the psychological and the political, and challenge the assumption that psychological and neurobiological sets of knowledge are inherently harmful, and opposed to feminism. They complexify the understandings of harm in relation to sexual violence, by broadening the lens on what is often understood in terms of (mental) health.

Suzanne Egan's chapter explores how psychiatric and psychological discourses are put to work in feminist sexual assault services in Australia. Egan explores the uses of the notion of trauma as a feminist practice. She examines the cohabitation of feminist analyses of violence as an issue of gendered power with the neuroscience of trauma. In rape crisis and sexual assault services, trauma-informed care has become synonymous with "best practice". Drawing on current policy documents, training manuals, industry research reports and worker interviews, this chapter examines the ways in which the neuroscience of trauma is put to work via its translation into specific policies, practices, and programmes. Egan documents the roles of psychiatric and psychology professionals in training workers in feminist services, and the uses to which these ideas and discourses are put by non-medical professionals. In her chapter, Stephanie Pache examines the construction of medical and psychiatric expertise behind sexual violence prevention programmes in Quebec. Her chapter nuances the depoliticising effect of psy-knowledge, and documents various uses of psy-knowledge in feminist movements. Still, as she shows, this knowledge can be used in "ambivalent" ways. Namely, the historical association of feminism, psy sciences and policy change raises epistemological and political issues, such as the use of psy sciences to promote prevention approaches that hinder the social and political causes of violence.

The final two chapters of this section highlight certain limitations of medical and psychiatric knowledge when applied to sexual violence, and present ways of thinking beyond a medicalised framing. They do so either by formulating models which account for the social and political roots of violence and victimisation, or by fostering knowledge informed by lived experience instead of medical aetiologies. Both chapters examine the gendered, racialised, and ableist construction of medical and psychiatric knowledge and power.

Andy Kaladelfos and Lisa Featherstone's chapter explores the construction of medical and psychiatric knowledge about child sexual abuse in Australia from the 1920s-1960s. The authors document the diffusion of medical and psychological terminologies and concepts beyond the medical sphere, notably in police technologies. They compare lawmakers' and state officials' perceptions of medical explanations of child sexual offences to the views of doctors and psy-experts, analysing their often-hostile exchanges about the value of medical testimony in criminal justice settings. This chapter calls the power of medicine and psychiatry into question. It shows how medicalised knowledge framed around "insanity" and the need for "social segregation" and "mental treatment" instead of imprisonment, corporal punishment, and capital punishment, was sometimes superseded by moral ideologies of sin or wrongdoing, and by eugenic discourses. Based on political debates, child sexual abuse prosecutions, judge's sentencing remarks, news reports and medical literature, the chapter highlights the limited influence of medical ideas amongst caregivers, experts and judges. Despite its influence, medical opinion was adapted and challenged in legal settings as well as in public perceptions and its framing of offending and prevention were not immune from racialised, gendered, and ableist framings.

Finally, Patsie Frawley highlights how contemporary medical knowledge about intellectual disability as a deficit contributes to violence and abuse. Drawing on narrative co-research with women with disabilities in Australia and New Zealand, the chapter documents how sexual ableism, deficit ways of thinking about women with disabilities have framed women with disabilities as sexually vulnerable. Ideas of vulnerability and their medicalised background are described as harmful and as a factor in the systemic abuse of people with disabilities. Indeed, congregate care and institutionalisation have been places of abuse. Against this backdrop, the chapter challenges the idea of inherent vulnerability and calls for a reframing of prevention of sexual violence against women and girls with disabilities that rejoins gender-based prevention efforts. Opposing this deficit focus—akin to "victim blaming"—Frawley's chapter presents an alternative model of disability violence and abuse that allows a systemic analysis. Stories of sexual violence and abuse occupy an important part of the chapter. Against the reduction to the single factor of disability, these stories centre individual, relational, community and societal factors accounting for the gendered ableist and systemic abuse experienced. Her contribution examines how knowledge which centre lived experience might help us to move beyond medicalised models, to reformulate understandings of sexual violence that account for the social elements contributing to victimisation.

The second section of this book sheds light on the uses of medical and forensic knowledge in sexual assault cases. How do health professionals interact with the legal system and how does medical evidence translate into legal categories? How do medical understandings of responses to sexual violence translate onto lived experience? In the articulation of medical and psychiatric knowledge in legal proceedings, social hierarchies and normative understandings of sexual violence and victimhood are brought to the fore. This section speaks to the ways in which medical and psychiatric knowledge functions within the legal realm. The chapters assert that forensic technologies and evidence gathering also need to be considered within their historical context: one in which Black women's bodies have been considered readily available for medical intervention, and where cooperation with carceral justice systems is actively encouraged. In doing so, the contributors challenge binary distinctions between truth and falsity, between what is known and unknown, and question how "just" justice systems really are.

This section demonstrates the power of medical and psychiatric evidence in sexual violence trials (Gotell 2002, 2008; Temkin 2002; Ellison 2009). Although such evidence is often presented as objective, these chapters reveal the various injustices incurred by medical and psychiatric evidence. Sameena Mulla and Heather Hlavka's chapter pertains to their ongoing work examining institutional responses to sexual assault in Milwaukee County Court, Wisconsin (Powell et al. 2017). In it, they demonstrate how expert knowledge from forensic nurses, medical personnel, and legal professionals both marks, and is marked by, hegemonic understandings of sexual violence, gender, and race. Throwing into sharp relief the historic racism of both the legal treatment of sexual violence, and historical understandings of obstetrics and gynaecology, they reveal with clarity the enduring influence of the racialising regimes of colonialism and chattel slavery. In their deft appraisal of these cases, they demonstrate that medical evidence is both produced by, and reproduces, harmful ideas about sexual violence at the nexus of race and gender, and hence, legal understandings of "normal" experiences of sexual violence.

In the following two chapters, the authors continue to question legalised understandings of "normal" experiences of sexual violence. Both chapters engage with the specific relationship between sleep and sexual violence, and how this is understood by the law. The second chapter, by Gethin Rees, Deborah White, and Natalie Wortley takes up the controversial case of Jade McCrossen-Nethercott in England and Wales. In 2017, Jade contacted the police to report that she had experienced sexual violence at an after-party in London, which had occurred while she was asleep. The controversy ensued when Jade's case was later dropped before progressing to trial, due to evidence suggesting that she suffered from "sexsomnia", and hence her assailant had a reasonable belief in consent on the night in question. The chief prosecutorial body in England and Wales have since apologised to Jade for their treatment of her case, but the authors dwell on what the history of the diagnosis of "sexsomnia" means for sexual violence cases more broadly. In doing so, they reveal the complexities around admitting expert scientific evidence in sexual violence cases, and some of the failures to regulate it.

In the third and final chapter in this section, Solveig Laugerud takes up the novel legal treatment of sexual violence cases in Norway. Although sexual violence trials commonly turn on the question of an individual's ability to resist an assault (commonly known as the "fight" or "flight" response), in Norway, the "freeze" response is additionally acknowledged as a legitimate response to sexual violence by the Criminal Justice System (Houge and Laugerud 2023). In this chapter, Laugerud examines how medical knowledge relating to the "freeze" response figures in the adjudication of sexual violence cases. In doing so, Laugerud takes up some of the themes discussed in the previous chapter, including the law's difficulty with categorising such states as sleep, intoxication, and in-between-states, which are conceptualised by Laugerud as "liminal hotspots". Laugerud's aim is to further conceptualise victims' responses to rape, and to continue her commitment to writing that calls into question how far the aftermath of sexual violence has been medicalised (Laugerud 2019).

Taken together, these chapters demonstrate the legal power of scientific evidence and medical understandings of sexual violence. In doing so, they additionally forge new ground into theorising forensic, carceral, and biomedical technologies of surveillance and discipline within the sexual violence field. Legal, medical, and psychiatric discourses concerning sexual violence are here powerfully shaped by a white, hegemonic, femininity, and a notion of trauma that demonstrates how the legitimacy of sexual violence testimony is adjudicated.

The volume's final section historicises medical and psychiatric approaches to sexual violence, providing essential context for the volume's broader discussion of questions of the production of knowledge and expertise in sexual assault cases. The historiography of gender-based violence in general, and of sexual violence in particular, has been growing since the turn towards women's and gender histories in the late twentieth century. Such work has provided essential insights into the social and cultural histories of sexual violence. There is not space here to do justice to the breadth of this work, but some key developments are worth noting. Second-wave feminist authors such as Susan Brownmiller

(1975) explored the ways in which rape was facilitated by societal power inequalities between men and women. Brownmiller's writing has been rightly critiqued for a lack of attention to intersectional dynamics, particularly the racialised valences of sexualised violence (Davis 1981; Crenshaw 1989; Bourke 2007, 2022), as well as for its failure to acknowledge the specific social, cultural, and historical contexts in which sexual violence occurs (Walker 2013; Bourke 2022). Sexual violence is not a transhistorical constant, but rather differs over space and time. In Joanna Bourke's formulation, "terror is always local" (2022, 3).

Historians, then, have explored these spatial and temporal contingencies, turning their attention to diverse aspects of sexual violence, from perceptions of rape (Clark 1987; Bourke 2007) to the evolution of the law in varied contexts (Hasday 2000; Saunders 2000; Rudolph 2000). Scholars have also examined the role of racialisation and of colonisation on sexual violence and its adjudication (Kolsky 2010; Shadle 2008; Thornberry 2019; Feimster 2009) and historicised conflict-related sexual violence (Branche and Virgili 2012; Mertens 2023; Keyse 2023). In relation to the intersection between the histories of sexual violence, medicine, and psychiatry, scholars have examined the historical uses of forensic evidence (Robertson 1998), as well as the uses of medical and psychiatric discourses in both constituting the figure of the sexual offender (Freedman 1987; Weston 2018) and understanding the emotional impacts of sexual violence on victims and survivors (Ruberg 2013; Bourke 2012). Other work has focused on the roles of particular medical professionals such as police surgeons and community health practitioners in identifying and responding to sexual violence (Beecher 2023; Bourke 2018). The chapters in this section contribute to this rich and burgeoning historiography.

Uncovering the traces of sexual violence from the archive is replete with challenges, as several historians navigating such sources have attested (Mertens 2023; Bridger and Hazan 2022). The first chapter in this section, by Joanna Zofia Spyra, engages directly with these methodological issues. Drawing on research conducted within the archives of *Ezras Noshim,* a community organisation assisting Jewish immigrant women and girls in interwar Argentina, Spyra explores how excavating the traces of sexual violence in community archives can provide broader perspectives than those found in the more "traditional" legal and medical sources favoured by historians of such violence. Spyra draws attention to the difficulties of applying concepts such as "sexual violence" to historical sources which do not explicitly or neatly categorise experiences as such. Through her excavation of the stories of women and girls experiencing sexual violence and exploitation in Buenos Aires in the mid-1930s, Spyra traces the ways in which pathologising medical discourses were used by non-medical organisations. Victims and survivors approaching *Ezras Noshim* for assistance could find their stories dismissed as indicators of mental instability, with consequences for their ability to access care and support. In navigating these stories, Spyra uses Miranda Fricker's (2007) concept of "epistemic injustice" to explore how women's knowledge of their circumstances and lived experiences were historically dismissed.

The following chapter, by Rhian Elinor Keyse, highlights the importance of historical context for understanding current challenges in responding to sexual violence. Taking as a starting point the obstacles to post-assault care and evidence gathering faced by victims and survivors of sexual assault in contemporary Kenya, Keyse argues that these issues have a longer historical trajectory and must be understood in the context of Kenya's settler colonial past. The chapter first explores the difficulties that women and girls faced in navigating colonial medico-legal structures, arguing that these barriers were rooted in the logics of colonial Kenya's racially stratified society. Underfunding of so-called "Native" medical facilities, and the prioritisation of white settler communities' needs in the development of colonial infrastructure hindered African women's access to medical care and forensic medical examinations in the aftermath of sexual assault. The chapter then explores the uses of medico-legal evidence in the colonial courtroom, arguing that medical "expertise" served to produce and reproduce gendered, classed, and racialised knowledge about victims and survivors of sexual violence.

In the volume's final chapter, George J. Severs deftly explores how understandings of sexual violence and consent influenced the responses of medical doctors working in medico-legal contexts to the emergence of the HIV test in mid-1980s Britain. Severs argues that the late 1980s saw a "crisis of consent", with the British government's "wartime response" to the HIV/AIDS epidemic contributing and responding to a climate of panic and anxiety, and undermining patients' rights to consent to medical testing. Severs demonstrates that this crisis was short-lived, and consent formed an important part of police surgeons' thinking about HIV testing. The evolution of such liberal responses to the pandemic was influenced by ideas about rape and sexual violence. However, the primacy of consent had its limitations which were thrown into sharp relief at the intersection between medicine and the criminal legal system. Severs demonstrates how, in coercive environments such as the prison or custody suite, medics were more likely to disregard patient consent than in other contexts such as the genitourinary clinic. By highlighting these nuances, this chapter contributes to an understanding of the tensions between medical care and coercion in carceral contexts.

**Funding** This work was supported by the Wellcome Trust (grant ID 205378/Z/16/Z), as part of the Sexual Harms and Medical Encounters project. The authors declare no competing interests.

## References

Basu, Koyel. 2024. Sexual Violence on Uyghurs: China's Conspiracy of 'Silence' in 21st Century's Greatest Holocaust. *International Journal of Human Rights and Constitutional Studies* 11: 62–76.

Beecher, Ruth. 2023. Children, Sexual Abuse and the Emotions of the Community Health Practitioner in England and Wales, 1970–2000. *Journal of the History of Medicine and Allied Sciences* 78: 365–380.

Berenstain, Nora. 2020. White Feminist Gaslighting. *Hypatia* 35: 733–758.

Bourke, Joanna. 2007. *Rape: A History From 1860 to the Present*. London: Virago.

Bourke, Joanna. 2012. Sexual Violence, Bodily Pain, and Trauma: A History. *Theory, Culture, and Society* 29: 25–51.

Bourke, Joanna. 2018. Police Surgeons and Victims of Rape: Cultures of Harm and Care. *Social History of Medicine* 31: 711–731.

Bourke, Joanna. 2022. *Disgrace: Global Reflections on Sexual Violence*. London: Reaktion Books.

Branche, Raphaëlle, and Fabrice Virgili, eds. 2012. *Rape in Wartime*. London: Palgrave Macmillan.

Bridger, Emily, and Erin Hazan. 2022. Surfeit and Silence: Sexual Violence in the Apartheid Archive. *African Studies* 83: 286–305.

Brownmiller, Susan. 1975. *Against Our Will: Men, Women, and Rape*. London: Secker and Warburg.

Burgess, Ann Wolbert, and Lynda Lyttle Holmstrom. 1974. Rape Trauma Syndrome. *American Journal of Psychiatry* 131: 981–986.

Busol, Kateryna. 2023. When the Head of State Makes Rape Jokes, His Troops Rape on the Ground: Conflict-Related Sexual Violence in Russia's Aggression Against Ukraine. *Journal of Genocide Research* 25: 279–314.

Butler, Judith. 1992. Contingent Foundations: Feminism and the Question of "Postmodernism." In *Feminists Theorise the Political*, ed. Judith Butler and Joan W. Scott, 3–21. New York: Routledge.

Clark, Anna. 1987. *Men's Violence, Women's Silence: Sexual Assault in England, 1770–1845*. London: Pandora.

Corrigan, Rose. 2013. *Up Against a Wall: Rape Reform and the Failure of Success*. New York: New York University Press.

Crenshaw, Kimberlé. 1989. Demarginalizing the Intersection of Race and Sex: A Black Feminist Critique of Antidiscrimination Doctrine, Feminist Theory, and Antiracist Politics. *University of Chicago Legal Forum* 139: 139–167.

Das, Veena. 2003. Trauma and testimony: Implications for political community. *Anthropological theory* 3, 3: 293–307.

Davis, Angela Y. 1981. *Women, Race, and Class*. New York: Random House.

Demeter, Márton. 2020. *Academic Knowledge Production and the Global South: Questioning Inequality and Underrepresentation*. Cham: Palgrave Macmillan.

Du Mont, Janice, and Deborah Parnis. 2000. Sexual Assault and Legal Resolution: Querying the Medical Collection of Forensic Evidence. *Medicine and Law* 19: 779–792.

Ellison, Louise. 2009. The Use and Abuse of Psychiatric Evidence in Rape Trials. *International Journal of Evidence & Proof* 13: 28–49.

Feimster, Crystal N. 2009. *Southern Horrors: Women and the Politics of Rape and Lynching*. Cambridge, MA: Harvard University Press.

Freedman, Estelle B. 1987. 'Uncontrolled Desires': The Response to the Sexual Psychopath, 1920–1960. *Journal of American History* 74: 83–106.

Fricker, Miranda. 2007. *Epistemic Injustice: Power and the Ethics of Knowing*. Oxford: Oxford University Press.

Goozee, Hannah. 2021. Decolonizing Trauma with Frantz Fanon. *International Political Sociology* 15: 102–120.

Gotell, Lise. 2002. The Ideal Victim, the Hysterical Complainant, and the Disclosure of Confidential Records: The Implications of the Charter for Sexual Assault Law. *Osgoode Hall Law Journal* 40: 251–293.

Gotell, Lise. 2008. Tracking Decisions on Access to Sexual Assault Complainants' Confidential Records: The Continued Permeability of Subsections 278.1-278.9 of the Criminal Code. *Canadian Journal of Women and the Law* 20: 111–54.

Hasday, Jill Elaine. 2000. Contest and Consent: A Legal History of Marital Rape. *California Law Review* 88: 1373–1505.

Herman, Judith Lewis. 1992. *Trauma and Recovery: The Aftermath of Violence - From Domestic Abuse to Political Terror*. New York: Basic Books.

Herman, Judith Lewis. 2015. *Trauma and Recovery: The Aftermath of Violence - From Domestic Abuse to Political Terror*, 2nd ed. New York: Basic Books.

Hlavka, Heather R., and Sameena Mulla. 2021. *Bodies in Evidence: Rape Victims, Forensic Nurses, and Sexual Assault Intervention.* New York: New York University Press.

Houge, Anette Bringedal, and Solveig Laugerud. 2023. "Unconscious or for Other Reasons Incapable of Resisting": (Un)Protected Sexual Assault Under Norwegian Criminal Law. *Violence Against Women.* https://doi.org/10.1177/10778012231181048.

Human Rights Watch. 2024. *"Khartoum Is Not Safe For Women!": Sexual Violence Against Women and Girls in Sudan's Capital.* New York: Human Rights Watch.

Keyse, Rhian Elinor. 2023. "A Very Sensitive Rwandan Woman": Sexual Violence, History, and Gendered Narratives in the Trial of Pauline Nyiramasuhuko at the International Criminal Tribunal for Rwanda, 2001–2011. *Women's History Review* 32: 1015–1039.

Kolsky, Elizabeth. 2010. "The Body Evidencing the Crime": Rape on Trial in Colonial India, 1860–1947. *Gender & History* 22: 109–130.

Lakshmi, Charan J. 2024. Challenges for Rape Survivors: Ban on Abortions in the USA. *Journal of Forensic Science and Medicine* 10: 163–164.

Laugerud, Solveig. 2019. Narrating the Harm of Rape: How Rape Victims Invoke Different Models of Psychological Trauma. *BioSocieties* 16: 22–40.

Lederer, Edith M. 2024. Red Cross Envoy: Congo Conflict Has Worsened With Sharp Increases in Sexual Violence and Wounded. *The Independent*, 27 June. https://www.independent.co.uk/news/congo-ap-red-cross-rwanda-united-nations-b2569710.html. Accessed on 10 September 2024.

Marsh, M., S. Purdin, and S. Navani. 2006. Addressing Sexual Violence in Humanitarian Emergencies. *Global Public Health* 1: 133–146.

Medie, Peace A., and Alice J. Kang. 2018. Power, Knowledge, and the Politics of Gender in the Global South. *European Journal of Politics and Gender* 1: 37–54.

Mertens, Charlotte. 2023. In the Ruins of Empire: Historicizing Sexual Violence in Congo. *International Feminist Journal of Politics* 25: 529–550.

Mulla, Sameena. 2014. *The Violence of Care: Rape Victims, Forensic Nurses, and Sexual Assault Intervention.* New York: New York University Press.

Nordstrom, Carolyn. 1996. Rape: Politics and Theory in War and Peace. *Australian Feminist Studies* 11: 147–162.

Office of the United Nations High Commissioner for Human Rights. 2024. *UN Experts Appalled by Reported Human Rights Violations Against Palestinian Women and Girls.* Office of the United Nations High Commissioner for Human Rights. https://www.ohchr.org/en/press-releases/2024/02/israel opt-un-experts-appalled-reported-human-rights-violations-against. Accessed on 10 September 2024.

Pande, Ishita. 2012. Coming of Age: Law, Sex, and Childhood in Late Colonial India. *Gender & History* 24: 205–230.

Phipps, Alison. 2020. *Me, Not You: The Trouble with Mainstream Feminism*. Manchester: Manchester University Press.

Powell, Amber Joy, Heather R. Hlavka, and Sameena Mulla. 2017. Intersectionality and Credibility in Child Sexual Assault Trials. *Gender and Society* 31: 457–480.

Quinlan, Andrea. 2017. *The Technoscientific Witness of Rape: Contentious Histories of Law, Feminism, and Forensic Science*. Toronto: University of Toronto Press.

Robertson, Stephen. 1998. Signs, Marks, and Private Parts: Doctors, Legal Discourses, and Evidence of Rape in the United States, 1823–1930. *Journal of the History of Sexuality* 8: 345–388.

Ruberg, Willemijn. 2013. Trauma, Body, and Mind: Forensic Medicine in Nineteenth-Century Dutch Rape Cases. *Journal of the History of Sexuality* 22: 85–104.

Rudolph, Julia. 2000. Rape and Resistance. Women and Consent in Seventeenth-century English Legal and Political Thought. *Journal of British Studies* 39: 157–184.

Saunders, Corinne. 2000. The Medieval Law of Rape. *King's Law Journal* 11: 19–48.

Shadle, Brett L. 2008. Rape in the Courts of Gusiiland, Kenya, 1940s–1960s. *African Studies Review* 51: 27–50.

Singh, Gagan Preet. 2021. Forensics, Body and State Power in South Asia: Recent Interventions and Their Importance. *History Compass* 19. https://doi.org/10.1111/hic3.12693.

Spurgas, Alyson K. 2021. Solidarity in Falling Apart: Toward a Crip, Collectivist, and Justice-Seeking Theory of Feminine Fracture. *Lateral* 10. https://doi.org/10.25158/l10.1.9.

Sweet, Paige. 2021. *The Politics of Surviving: How Women Navigate Domestic Violence and its Aftermath*. Oakland, CA: University of California Press.

Temkin, Jennifer. 2002. *Rape and the Legal Process*. Oxford: Oxford University Press.

Thornberry, Elizabeth. 2019. *Colonizing Consent: Rape and Governance in South Africa's Eastern Cape*. Cambridge: Cambridge University Press.

UNAIDS. 2022. *Dangerous Inequalities: World AIDS Day Report 2022*. Geneva: Joint United Nations Programme on HIV/AIDS.

UN Women. 2020. *Covid-19 and Ending Violence Against Women and Girls*. New York: UN Women.

Walker, Garthine. 2013. Sexual Violence and Rape in Europe, 1500–1750. In *The Routledge History of Sex and the Body, 1500 to the Present*, ed. Sarah Toulalan and Kate Fisher, 429–443. New York: Routledge.

Weston, Janet. 2018. *Medicine, the Penal System, and Sexual Crimes in England, 1919–1960s: Diagnosing Deviance*. London: Bloomsbury.

# Psycho-Medical Expertise in Question

# Exploring Trauma as Feminist Praxis in the Australian Field of Sexual Assault Service Provision

*Suzanne Egan*

## 1 Introduction

Trauma is not an entirely new concept to feminism; however, the uptake of trauma in its present iteration—as part of a formalised psychiatric nomenclature—within feminist work against sexual violence is contentious. Within feminist scholarship, 'trauma talk' (Marecek 1999) is often represented as symptomatic of a decline in feminist politics and influence, evidence of the medicalisation of sexual assault, an incursion that reduces a social and political issue to a problem of individual mental health (Burstow 2005; Gavey and Schmidt 2011; O'Dell 2003; Whittier 2009; Wilkin and Hillock 2014). However, in community settings such as rape crisis and sexual assault organisations, the trauma model has become synonymous with this field of work. Organisations are typically prompted as taking a 'trauma-informed' approach or as 'trauma specialists', with terms such as 'sexual assault counselling' and 'trauma counselling' used interchangeably in some settings. Rather than antithetical, the trauma

S. Egan (✉)
School of Social Sciences, Western Sydney University, Sydney, NSW, Australia
e-mail: s.egan@westernsydney.edu.au



R. E. Keyse et al. (eds.), *Sexual Violence in Medicine and Psychiatry*, Genders and Sexualities in History,
https://doi.org/10.1007/978-3-032-10800-5_2

model and trauma work are often understood as integral to feminist work against sexual violence (Brensell 2022; Egan 2019, 2020).

This chapter focuses on the Australian sexual assault services sector, drawing on interviews conducted with sexual assault workers to explore their experiences of and views on the possibilities of a relationship between feminism, trauma, and neuroscience. It is an endeavour undertaken in the spirit of 'critical friendship' (Rose and Abi-Rached 2013), one which neither aims to dismiss the concerns raised in feminist scholarship nor to unreservedly embrace the trauma model. Rather, I am interested in exploring what the 'psy' sciences (medicine, psychiatry, psychology) look like when dispersed from the clinic and the laboratory and taken up in a specific applied context. The chapter in no way aims to discount or ignore the very real harms that medical and psychiatric knowledges and practices can do, and have done, to survivors of sexual violence, both within their own distinctive discursive frameworks and when enmeshed with deeply held and deeply problematic cultural and social beliefs around sexuality, gender, and race. However, the chapter does seek to problematise the conventional binary that positions medicine and the biological sciences as inherently harmful and in opposition to feminism, such that the only available engagement for feminist scholarship becomes 'the well-worn path of critique' (Alaimo and Hekman 2008, 4). I am interested in what seemingly problematic ideas can look like and be used, adopted and adapted, in specific situations and contexts (Müller and Kenney 2021). Indeed, as Müller and Kenney's (2021) recent ethnographic research on the biological framing of early life adversity and trauma-informed practice in a U.S. educational setting highlight, it is in such local situated contexts that we can most often see the specificity of how a discourse is interpreted and the varied applications of seemingly problematic ideas.

In what follows, I provide a synopsis of key concerns raised in feminist scholarship about the 'turn' to trauma, then move on to an overview of sexual assault service provision in Australia before turning to explore the ways in which sexual assault workers mobilise trauma in a way that 'fits' with their feminist counselling practices. First, though, a note on the concept of trauma, a term that has become so ubiquitous that it is often not seen as requiring explanation (Becker-Blease 2017; Fassin and Rechtman 2009).

## 2 A Note on the Concept of Trauma

In a general sense, the concept of psychological trauma rests on the premise that while some harmful experiences—sexual assault, for example—may not result in physical injury, they have profoundly injurious psychological and emotional effects on the individual. While the effects of physical trauma to the body are typically visible, a broken bone as the result of a fall or an open wound, the effects of psychological trauma are less visible, their marks left internally on the psyche of the individual.

In more formal terms, psychological trauma, in the form of post-traumatic stress disorder (PTSD) has been recognised as a psychiatric diagnosis since 1980 when it was first included in the *Diagnostic and Statistical Manual of Mental Disorders* (third edition, *DSM-III*) of the American Psychiatric Association (Young 1995). While the diagnostic criteria for PTSD have undergone some changes since that time (Pai et al. 2017; Young 1995), the core features remain consistent. In summary, an individual experiencing PTSD typically cycles between being overwhelmed with intrusive memories of the abuse, which may take the form of nightmares, flashbacks, sensations, or images and working to shut down and avoid these distressing memories, and avoiding any external reminders that could trigger these memories. The person often lives in a state of physiological arousal that may show as hyper alertness, a sense of being on guard, as startling easily, and/or difficulties with concentration, coupled with feelings of shame, guilt, or self-blame (American Psychiatric Association 2013; Herman 2015).

Complex trauma or complex PTSD, as the name suggests, denotes a more complex and diffuse set of effects associated with ongoing and repeated abuse and was first outlined by the American feminist and psychiatrist Judith Herman in her influential text *Trauma and Recovery: The Aftermath of Violence—From Domestic Abuse to Political Terror* (1992). While Herman was one of the first to propose that PTSD, a diagnosis initially associated with war veterans, encapsulated the experiences of victims of gendered violence, she also pointed to its limitations in capturing the more pervasive effects of abuse experienced in childhood, particularly child sexual abuse. Herman suggested that because early trauma adversely affects the child's psychological, emotional, and cognitive development, the effects are experienced into adulthood. Herman (1992) focused on the pejorative label of borderline personality disorder

(BPD), arguing that the rates of childhood abuse in the histories of such patients suggested that their 'symptoms' were not inherent personality flaws but rather should be understood as the ongoing effects of early trauma. While complex trauma (or C-PTSD) is not a specific diagnostic category in the *DSM*, it is widely recognised in psychological and trauma literature as a clinically recognised condition (see, for example, Courtois and Ford 2009; Kezelman and Stavropolous 2019). Complex trauma includes the effects encapsulated by PTSD as well as an additional set of effects that include difficulties in interpersonal relationship, self-harm and suicidality, and pervasive feelings of worthlessness and shame (Herman 2015; Karatzias and Levendosky 2019).

Increasingly, understandings of trauma and traumatic reactions have become informed by neuroscience or what Rose and Abi-Rachid (2013) refer to as the 'brain sciences'—for example, the idea that traumatic memory is encoded in a different part of the brain to normal memory and because of this is recalled in sensory rather than in verbal form (van der Kolk 2015). The development of new technologies such as functional magnetic resonance imaging (fMRI) has enabled researchers to begin charting the effects of traumatic experiences on the neurochemistry and anatomy of the brain (Stark et al. 2015). For example, research using fMRI scans has shown that sensory reminders of the abuse trigger brain activity that in turn results in physiological reactions in the body: the increase in adrenaline and cortisol, the elevated blood pressure and heart rate (van der Kolk 2015).

## 3 Feminist Concerns About the Uptake of Trauma

Internationally, the adoption of trauma models and frameworks in rape crisis and sexual assault service settings has been a source of some concern in feminist scholarship and writing. While the arguments and critiques are nuanced, they are underpinned by some common themes. First, much of the concern appears centred on the uptake of formal diagnostic categories such as PTSD and the use of the attendant trauma models and therapeutic interventions that have been developed based on these diagnostic categories. Often, there is a distinction drawn between the way in which feminists in the 1970s and 1980s used the concept of trauma, metaphorically for injury to the psyche versus the contemporary formalisation of trauma as a scientifically and medically based set of symptoms and effects (see, for example, Haaken and Lamb 2000; Levett 2003;

Marecek 1999; Whittier 2009). Second, and leading from this, is the concern that contemporary trauma discourse with its emphasis on diagnostic frameworks medicalises sexual assault, reducing a political and social issue to one of individual mental health (Lamb 1999; Mardorossian 2002; Marecek 1999). Indeed, in some commentary, the dominance of 'trauma talk' (Marecek 1999) in sexual assault organisations is attributed to a decline in feminist activism and the imposition of professionalised therapeutic interventions (Cvetkovich 2003; Stark 2007). A particular concern is the positioning of victims within a deficit discourse in which they become characterised as vulnerable and in need of care rather than as agentic survivors of a structural form of gendered violence. (Burstow 2005; Wilkin and Hillock 2014). For example, Burstow (2005) argues that the 'symptoms' associated with the diagnostic category of PTSD should be understood as survival strategies rather than as symptoms of a mental health problem that needs to be fixed. The argument that Burstow pursues is not that the concept of psychological trauma and its attendant effects be abandoned as a framework for understanding the effects of sexual violence. Rather the key 'symptoms' of PTSD are retained but removed from their psychiatric nosology through the reframing as signifiers of strength and survival.

The uptake of a form of knowledge based in medicine, psychiatry, and psychology does seem a curious development given that much of the impetus for setting up feminist rape crisis collectives across Western countries during the 1970s and 1980s was the poor treatment of victims by hospitals and the medical establishment (Carmody 1995; Carmody and Carrington 2000; Loney-Howes 2020). However, feminism, understood as an intersection of theoretical perspectives and political practices, has had, and continues to have, a complex, if 'uneasy', relationship with the psy disciplines, both disavowing and at times simultaneously appropriating and adapting these knowledges for its own use (Crook 2018; Germon 2009; Ruck et al. 2022). The term 'psy disciplines' is used to encapsulate disciplines such as psychology, psychiatry, psychotherapy, and psychoanalysis and to denote their increasing power and authority in explaining social concerns (Ruck et al. 2022). The related process of psychologisation refers to the ways in which the discourse of the psy disciplines penetrates other social fields and/or shapes everyday feeling, experience, and action (Ruck et al. 2022, 270).

Ruck et al.'s (2022) recent research on the psychologisation of the second wave women's movement in the United States and German-speaking countries has drawn attention to the ways in which radical feminists both rejected traditional psychological approaches as contributing to women's oppression *and* drew on key psychological concepts in the development of consciousness raising (CR), a political practice that, it could be argued, has come to signify second wave feminist political activism. Often signified via the slogan 'the personal is political', CR approached women's personal transformation as a conduit to broader social and cultural transformation.

As Ruck et al.'s (2022) careful and detailed research lays out, the feminists who developed CR were highly critical of the focus on individual responsibility that underpinned psychoanalysis and traditional forms of therapy and, particularly in the case of psychoanalysis, viewed them as disciplines grounded in belief systems that contributed to women's oppression. Yet their work highlights the extent to which the personal transformation phases of CR were grounded in such psychological concepts and practices. For example, in the United States, context CR groups implicitly drew on the psychoanalytic concept of defence mechanisms to explain why some women may resist consciousness raising—ideas that included identifying with and idealising the oppressor and finding justifications for their behaviour. In other instances, the uptake was more explicit. For example, Viennese feminist activists, who had often trained in psychotherapeutic methods, drew on these methods and included elements of gestalt therapy, as developed by medical practitioner and psychoanalyst Fritz Perls, bioenergetic therapy, as developed by medical practitioner and psychotherapist Alexander Lowen, and transactional analysis, which originated with psychiatrist Eric Berne (Ruck et al. 2022).

Through their detailed archival work, Ruck et al. (2022) carefully unpack the tensions and complexities in how psy expert discourse was taken up by feminists through an, at times, contradictory interpellation of critique, adaptation, and adoption. As they emphasise, the way in which feminist activists practised self-awareness was a result of their critique of psychology, but, although not always acknowledged, it was psychology nevertheless—because it was a form of CR that had already been refracted through the lens of psychologisation. Moreover, they draw attention to the tensions that existed within radical feminism from the early days (i.e., early 1970s) that CR could privilege well-being and personal transformation over radical social change. While CR encouraged women to understand the social and political origins of their individual experiences, this was underpinned by the expectation that such personal transformation would provide them with the impetus for involvement in collective political action and agitation for social change.

I find these to be significant observations given that second-wave feminist activism often appears as the measure against which contemporary feminist work is found lacking. It suggests that concerns about the influence of psy expertise, individualisation, and loss of political focus significantly predates current concerns about the 'turn' to trauma. Indeed, while the rise of therapeutic interventions is often juxtaposed against activist work, Ruck et al. (2022) draw attention to an alternative body of work, suggesting that social movements play a key role in the diffusion of the psy disciplines into social fields and everyday life. Overall, their work highlights the complexity in the way psy knowledge has been taken up in feminist work; while there can certainly be tensions, there are also productive possibilities that do not necessarily equate to depoliticisation or a decline in feminist influence.

## 4 The Australian Sexual Assault Services Sector

Like most Western nations, rape crisis and sexual assault services in Australia emerged from the second wave feminist movements of the 1970s and 1980s and over time have moved from grassroots to more professionalised and formalised organisational structures (see, for example, Beres et al. 2009; Brensell 2022). As an example, the Sydney Rape Crisis Collective (SRCC) was initially run by a feminist collective, both offering 24-hour crisis telephone support to individual victims and agitating for broader social change via political campaigns and protests. However, the SRCC also actively sought government funding almost from its inception in 1974, and over time, like most community-based sexual assault organisations in Australia, moved to a management structure and employment of paid counsellors with formal qualifications rather than volunteers (Egan 2020).[1] Currently known as Full Stop Australia, the organisation continues to provide crisis telephone, online support,

[1] This early move to actively seeking government funding is typical of the community-based, sometimes referred to as grassroots, organisations in Australia. As an example, one of the reasons that the incest collectives in New South Wales (NSW) formed a network, the Incest Survivors Network (ISN), in the early 1980s was to lobby for the funding that

and face-to-face counselling, runs a survivor advocate programme, and is involved in advocacy and prevention work (Full Stop Australia n.d.).

In the current Australian context, sexual assault services are a state rather than federal government responsibility, which means there is some local variation across the states in how sexual assault services sectors are organised. Generally, however, there is a combination of government services that are usually part of the health services sectors and based on either community health centres or hospital and non-government organisation (NGO) services that may be 'stand alone' rape crisis or child sexual assault centres or incorporated into larger services such as a women's health centres.[2] For example, in the state of New South Wales (NSW) where I conducted my research, there is a network of approximately 70 sexual assault services located in community health centres and hospitals within the public health system, together with a network of NGO child sexual assault services, as well as Full Stop Australia. Whether based in the government or community sector, sexual assault services continue to be involved in community education and prevention work, though their core daily work centres on providing crisis and ongoing counselling support to victims. In addition, one of the roles of the NSW Health sexual assault services is to coordinate the medical response to victims. This generally means that the service manager, or a designated crisis coordinator, ensures that doctors as well as counsellors are rostered on the 24-hour crisis service, while for individual counsellors, it means supporting the victim through the medical examination process, including supporting the person in deciding if they will undergo a medical examination (Egan 2020; NSW Health 2020).

Despite the formalisation of service provision and the attendant policies and processes, feminism continues to hold an authoritative position in sexual assault services. Indeed, as I have laid out in detail elsewhere,

the NSW state government was making available to organisations via the newly formed Child Sexual Assault policy (Carmody 1995).

[2] The combination of government and non-government services can be traced to the form that second wave feminism took in Australia at the time services originated. While many feminists were involved in 'grassroots organisations and activism' others often referred to as 'femocrats' worked for change from within the state bureaucracy. As an example, a well-known Australian feminist and eventual academic, the late Professor Moira Carmody, oversaw the development of the first child sexual assault policy in NSW that saw the rollout of child sexual assault services in both government and nongovernment settings across the state in the mid-1980s (Carmody 1995).

feminist knowledge/s of 'what sexual assault is' and why it happens both underpins worker practices and is embedded through the most basic element of service provision (Egan 2019, 2020). While there are nuances, a feminist analysis of sexual violence can be briefly encapsulated as an analysis of gendered power and violence in which the experiences of the individual (survivor) are understood through the broader patriarchal social structures that produce normative heterosexuality (Mason 2002). In the applied context of Australian sexual assault organisations, this analysis articulates into 'taken for granted' practices such as locating responsibility with the perpetrator of the abuse, in an attunement to the types of social beliefs and cultural practices that produce self-blame and in the capacity to locate individual experiences of sexual victimisation in the broader social and structural context (Egan 2020).

At the same time, sexual assault workers in the sector have been 'early adopters' of the neuroscience of trauma. For example, trauma experts such as John Briere and Bessel van der Kolk have been conducting training workshops in Australia since the late 1990s, with their research used to inform the professional development training and workshops provided to sexual assault practitioners (Egan 2024). At the time I began working in the NSW sexual assault services sector in the late 1990s, Judith Herman's (1997, 2001) trauma model was firmly entrenched in training and practice. Often referred to back then as 'the bible', her influential text, *Trauma and Recovery*, is both an explicitly feminist text and grounded in the psychology of PTSD. Herman's focus on psychological, emotional, and physical safety assisted me and my co-workers in being able to respond usefully to the often very concrete issues for which clients sought counselling. Equally important, Herman's emphasis on belief and support as feminist political practice as well as the clear analysis of the structural patriarchal underpinnings of sexual abuse and domestic violence helped us to better understand and situate our work, which on a daily basis typically focused on counselling work with individuals, as a legitimate form of feminist work.[3] In this context, the then emerging work on

[3] On my part, it is probably worth explaining that my university-based feminist and gender studies had been a 'heady' and at times confusing mix of post-structural feminist theorising coupled with a particular version of feminist social work in which counselling and working with individuals was positioned as 'not quite feminism' unless accompanied by more visible activist work. Both the highly theoretical and the firmly activist I found unsatisfactory in providing a useful grounding for the realities of my day-to-day work. This

the neuroscience of trauma (see, for example, van der Kolk 2000, 2004) provided an additional source of knowledge that helped us better understand some of the issues, such as flashbacks and dissociation, that the people I was working with often experienced and which underscored the importance of Herman's focus on safety as foundational to trauma work.

Over time, what could be seen as worker- or practice-led approaches[4] have been taken up at the organisational and policy level, resulting in the production of a range of 'trauma-focused' and 'trauma-informed' policy and related documents. These documents include governance documents such as the NSW Health sexual assault policy (2020) and best practice documents and assessment protocols (e.g., Hegarty et al. 2017; Kezelman and Stavropolous 2019, 2020) and assessment protocols. This formalisation of practice into policy and governance documents is a significant development, an indicator of the authoritative position and acceptance of the trauma model in sexual assault work (Gavey 2018). As an example, the previous NSW Health sexual assault policy and procedure manual that guided service delivery until 2020 made almost no mention of trauma. By contrast, the current manual (NSW Health 2020) contains extensive material on PTSD, on specific therapeutic trauma models, and on research focused on the neuroscience of trauma. This shift is reflective of the increasing adoption of trauma-informed practice as policy and practice guidelines across a range of systems including child protection, juvenile justice, mental health, and education over the last decade (Becker-Blease 2017). However, while policies and governance documents do influence practice, policy can be subverted or even ignored and, at a minimum, is subject to interpretation and local reworking as it articulates through practice.

Consequently, the discussion that follows centres on the accounts of the sexual assault practitioners I interviewed as part of a larger project on feminist knowledge practices in the sexual assault services sector in the state of NSW (Egan 2019, 2020). I focus first on their reflections

is a pity as it continued the unhelpful dichotomy and to some extent conflict between feminists working inside and those who work outside the academy.

[4] By worker- or practice-led approaches, I am referring to instances where what practitioners (those on the frontline) are doing and often have been doing for some time precedes the formalisation of those practices into policy guidelines and frameworks that guide service provision. It is something of an inversion of the policy–practice relationship in which, in social policy analysis, policies are often positioned as framing or driving on-the-ground practices.

on the increasing influence of trauma and then explore some of the ways in which practitioners engage with neuroscientific theories of trauma to support their counselling practices.

## 5 Sexual Assault Worker Reflections on Trauma as Feminist Praxis

Through the interviews, sexual assault practitioners used the space afforded to provide thoughtful and nuanced critical reflections, situating their own practices in broader trends and changes in the Australian sexual assault services sector. Practitioners who had extensive work histories in the sector consistently identified the increasing influence of trauma, sometimes articulated as the 'trauma model' but most often simply as 'trauma', as one of the major changes in their own understanding of sexual assault as well as across the sector more generally. Newer or less experienced practitioners typically identified trauma and the trauma model as the area they felt had been most important for them to gain an in-depth, applied understanding of when starting in their positions.

However, there was a keen awareness of the apparent incongruousness of a field of practice typically understood as 'a child of the feminist movement' (Interview Text No. 5) to actively engaging with concepts, research, and ideas based on medicine and psychiatry. As this practitioner highlights, reflecting on the changes she has observed over time,

> In the early days we would not have dared talk to male psychiatrists about how to work with women survivors of sexual abuse. It was very polarised. A mainstream medical model and a feminist model would have been very critical of each other. (Interview Text No. 17; Egan 2020)

And yet it is the work of the psychiatrists and psychologists with reputations as trauma researchers and specialists that is being used across this sector, including John Briere, Bessel van der Kolk, Colin Ross, and Judith Herman.[5] As discussed, their ideas and the models associated with them are incorporated through much of the ongoing learning and development training provided to sexual assault workers and were referred to frequently

[5] While a key figure in the feminist movement, Herman was also a trained psychiatrist, a fact that remains evident through each of the editions of her pioneering text *Trauma and Recovery* (1992, 1997, 2001, 2015).

across the interviews. Indeed, it was 'the neurobiology stuff' (Interview Text No. 27) that was often identified by practitioners as having the most utility in supporting their existing feminist practices.

Taking up the thread of the narrative, another practitioner reflects on the fears about pathologising victims of sexual assault that have run through the sector from its inception. In response to my follow-up question about the source of this concern, she explains,

> Well, I suppose, the medical model of victims are victims and sexual assault leaves them incapacitated, I suppose. I think, with this neurobiology stuff, it's sort of – it does recognise that there is some real harm that has happened to someone to their bodies, to their beings, but it's important not to buy too much into that as well, because people also have agency … it still doesn't leave the person without any control, as acted upon. (Interview Text No. 27; Egan 2020)

Here we can see a certain wariness about engaging with 'this neurobiology stuff', about the potential for 'buying into' a medical model that positions victims in deficit terms as somehow 'incapacitated' and 'acted upon'. Present too, though, is a consideration of the usefulness of recognising the embodied harms of trauma—the effect on their bodies and beings—along with mobilisation of a narrative about agency, control, and capacity to survive.

The following explanation of the effects of trauma on the brain traumatic memory is illustrative of the idea's practitioners used through the interviews. It is also typical of the type of representation of trauma provided across the various training workshops and programmes routinely undertaken by practitioners as part of their ongoing on the job learning and training.

> The parts of the brain that are most affected following a traumatic event are the imagery parts of the brain that are actually highlighted in – the chemical produced through PTSD shuts down the cognitive functions and the verbal functions but provides more stimulation and a greater amount to the imagery side, which is why flashbacks and nightmares are such a powerful part of post-traumatic stress disorder. … The brain fundamentally doesn't know the difference between what it imagines and what is. The brain will still – so a flashback can be experienced as – that it's actually happening – the body has the same reaction. (Interview Text No. 29; Egan 2020)

This is an account clearly influenced by and drawing on the neuroscience of trauma and traumatic memory. What is important, though, I would argue, is not so much the recourse to neurobiological representations of the trauma but how it is used and the types of practices it supports. As Müller and Kenney (2021) argue, drawing on Pickersgill (2018), biosocial narratives—of which neuroscience is a part—are 'neither inherently liberatory nor inherently oppressive' (1254) but rather can be used to support a range of different practices and political positions.

For example, the practitioner above went on to explain how she used this understanding of traumatic memory to work with victim/survivors to assist them, to understand experiences such as flashbacks or dissociation, which can be frightening and disorienting experiences over which the person feels very little control (Brison 2002). Such an understanding is a precursor to working with the person to regain a sense of control over their emotional, bodily, and psychological responses. 'It helps the person to understand what's going on and become more able to take charge of themselves again' (Interview Text No. 27). This might be grounding exercises such attention to the breath or working with the person at their own pace to slowly gain some control over the distressing images (Interview Text No. 29). Briere and Scott (2015) refer to this as 'titrating' or slowing the traumatic responses (emotional, physiological, and psychological) so the person moves from a state of overwhelm to regulation and integration. A key element in this trauma model and which was highlighted by practitioners was the focus on 'going with the client at their pace and their time in a sense and [knowing] that they will be the expert on [this]' (Interview Text No. 29). Indeed, the 'symptoms' of trauma, the oscillation between reactivation and avoidance of traumatic memory, are approached by Briere and Scott (2015) not as a pathology or as deficits to be fixed but as an inherent attempt to heal from the trauma.

Running through the practitioner narratives are accounts of how trauma and the neuroscience of trauma are actively and knowingly mobilised in ways that are compatible with feminist counselling practices and which the following interview excerpt has been selected to illustrate. In this interview excerpt, the practitioner provides a thoughtful account of how she brings together her structural gendered analysis of sexual violence with Briere's trauma model. As she reflects, it is about 'being able to pull out' whatever is needed in the moment. In some situations, this means a very deliberate and explicit exploration of the dynamics of gendered power and abuse, and at others, it is using the trauma-based skills and knowledge to alleviate the distressing embodied harms of traumatic violence:

> So, if that person is really struggling with 'I don't understand why I'm sitting at work, nothing's reminding me of this and then I get this flashback', then you pull in more on Briere's stuff. If I'm working with the woman I was describing before, who had a lifetime of sexual assault, she's losing her job from a very high-powered role as a woman. She wanted to talk about the attack and felt like 'was he trying to bring me down because I was more senior to him'. So then, I'm really drawing on the feminist ideas more strongly, plus some trauma. So, it's that thing of being able to pull out whatever [you need] at the time. (Interview Text No. 23; Egan 2020)

In the above excerpt, the practitioner draws attention to the importance of being guided by the issues that the client brings to counselling and which she wants to talk about. When her client, who was subject to sexual abuse in her work context, wanted to talk about the overt abuse of power of her abuser, 'the wanting to bring me down', the counsellor drew on a feminist analysis of gendered power, its operation in the corporate world, and articulation through the sexual abuse perpetrated by the woman's work colleague. When it is the flashbacks that seem to come out of nowhere, then the counsellor is guided by Briere and work on traumatic memory.

## 6 Concluding Discussion

Through this chapter, I have used a specific applied context (Müller and Kenney 2021) to explore the ways in which trauma and the neurobiological framing of trauma is understood and mobilised by workers employed in Australian sexual assault organisations. The exploration has been informed by an interest in considering trauma as compatible with rather than as antithetical to feminist practice. I have focused specifically on counselling practices both because it is core to the role played by workers in sexual assault services and because it is the intervention that has attracted the most concern in feminist scholarship on the uptake of trauma.

There are three key points that I want to highlight. First, the reflexivity and knowingness displayed in sexual assault workers' accounts of their engagement with trauma discourse are noteworthy. Rather being either imposed or unknowingly absorbed as simply 'the way things are done', the uptake of trauma was an active change in their own practice experiences, as well as a change they had observed over time across the sector. Practitioners were keenly aware of the centrality of feminism in the origins and development of their own services and the sector more broadly as well as cognisant of the conflictual history and potential problems of engaging with knowledge based on medicine and psychiatry. Indeed, some had worked in rape crisis organisations long enough to have observed and been part of the shifts and turns from outright dismissal to cautious engagement. In this way, what appears in their accounts is not so much the cycling between the disavowal and adoption unpacked by Ruck et al. (2022) in their analysis of radical feminism and CR but the adoption of a critically reflexive stance that encompasses a wary if optimistic adoption.

Second, and related, concern about not buying into or replicating a medical model that positions sexual assault victims as incapacitated was tempered by consideration of what had proved useful about the neuroscience of trauma. This included helping the practitioners to work with the embodied effects of trauma, with the types of concerns with which their clients often sought counselling, including distressing flashbacks to the abuse, the constant triggers and feeling of 'being on alert', and the emotional and affective toll of those reactions. Finally, this translates into working with the survivor in a way that can assist her in making sense of her reactions and understanding the expected and 'normal' responses to the traumatic experience of sexual violence. The problem is not her reactions but the violent acts to which she has been subject. Used in this way, trauma discourse can be used as a tool in a feminist practice in which working with the client at their own pace in order to regain a sense of control in the aftermath of a disempowering and abusive experience remains central.

**Funding and Competing Interests** The author does not have any funding or competing interests to declare.

## References

Alaimo, Stacy, and Susan Hekman. 2008. Introduction: Emerging Models of Materiality in Feminist Theory. In *Material Feminisms*, ed. S. Alaimo and S. Hekman, 1–19. Bloomington, IN: Indiana University Press.

American Psychiatric Association. 2013. *Diagnostic and Statistical Manual of Mental Disorders*, 5th ed. Washington DC: American Psychiatric Publishing.

Becker-Blease, Kathryn. 2017. As the World Becomes Trauma-Informed, Work to Do. *Journal of Trauma and Dissociation* 18: 131–138.

Beres, Melanie, Barbaran Crow, and Lise Gotell. 2009. The Perils of Institutionalization in Neoliberal Times: Results of a National Survey of Canadian Sexual Assault and Rape Crisis Centres. *Canadian Journal of Sociology* 34: 135–164.

Brensell, Ariane. 2022. *Contextualized Trauma Work*. https://kontextualisierte-traumaarbeit.de/. Accessed on 6 September 2024.

Briere, John N., and Catherine Scott. 2015. *Principles of Trauma Therapy: A Guide to Symptoms, Evaluation, and Treatment*, 2nd ed. Los Angeles: SAGE.

Brison, Susan. 2002. *Aftermath: Violence and the Remaking of a Self*. Princeton, NJ: Princeton University Press.

Burstow, Bonnie. 2005. A Critique of Posttraumatic Stress Disorder and the DSM. *Journal of Humanistic Psychology* 45: 429–445.

Carmody, Moira. 1995. *Sites of Struggle: The Development of Social Policy Surrounding Rape and Sexual Assault Services in New South Wales, Australia*. Unpublished PhD thesis, University of New South Wales Sydney.

Carmody, Moira, and Kerry Carrington. 2000. Preventing Sexual Violence? *Australian & New Zealand Journal of Criminology* 33: 341–361.

Courtois, Christine A., and Julian D. Ford. 2009. *Treating Complex Traumatic Stress Disorders: An Evidence-Based Guide*. New York: Guilford Press.

Crook, Sarah. 2018. The Women's Liberation Movement, Activism, and Therapy at the Grassroots, 1968–1985. *Women's History Review* 27: 1152–1168. https://doi.org/10.1080/09612025.2018.1450611.

Cvetkovich, Ann. 2003. *An Archive of Feelings: Trauma, Sexuality, and Lesbian Public Cultures*. Durham, NC: Duke University Press.

Egan, Suzanne. 2019. Excavating Feminist Knowledges and Practices in the Field of Sexual Assault Service Provision: An Australian Case Study. *Women's Studies International Forum* 74: 169–178. https://doi.org/10.1016/j.wsif.2019.04.001.

Egan, Suzanne. 2020. *Putting Feminism to Work: Theorising Sexual Violence, Trauma, and Subjectivity*. Cham: Palgrave Macmillan. https://doi.org/10.1007/978-3-030-22109-6.

Egan, Suzanne. 2024. Deploying Rose, and Abi-Rached to 'Make Sense' of the Rise of the 'Brain Sciences' in the Field of Violence Against Women. In *Using Social Theory in Higher Education*, eds. R. Low, S. Egan and A. Bell, 77–90. Cham: Palgrave Macmillan.

Fassin, Didier, and Richard Rechtman. 2009. *The Empire of Trauma: An Inquiry Into the Condition of Victimhood*, trans. R. Gomme. Princeton: Princeton University Press.

Full Stop Australia. n.d. *Homepage*. https://fullstop.org.au/. Accessed on 5 January 2024.

Gavey, Nicola. 2018. *Just Sex?: The Cultural Scaffolding of Rape* (2nd ed.), Oxford: Routledge.

Gavey, Nicola, and Johana Schmidt. 2011. 'Trauma of Rape' Discourse: A Double-Edged Template for Everyday Understandings of the Impact of Rape? *Violence against Women* 17: 433–456.

Germon, Jennifer. 2009. *Gender: A Genealogy of an Idea*. Basingstoke: Palgrave Macmillan.

Haaken, Janice, and Sharon Lamb. 2000. The Politics of Child Sexual Abuse Research. *Society* 37: 7–14.

Hegarty, Kelsey, Laura Tarzia, Susan Rees, Alyssha Fooks, Kirsty Forsdike, Delanie Woodlock, Lisa Simpson, Clare McCormack, and Sue Amanatidis. 2017. *Women's Input Into a Trauma-Informed Systems Model of Care in Health Settings (The WITH Study) Final report*. Sydney: ANROWS Horizons.

Herman, Judith. 1992. *Trauma and Recovery: The Aftermath of Violence – From Domestic Abuse to Political Terror*. New York: Basic Books.

Herman, Judith. 1997. *Trauma and Recovery: The Aftermath of Violence – From Domestic Abuse to Political Terror*. New York: Basic Books.

Herman, Judith Lewis. 2001. *Trauma and Recovery. From Domestic Abuse to Political Terror*. London: Pandora.

Herman, Judith Lewis. 2015. *Trauma and Recovery: The Aftermath of Violence – From Domestic Abuse to Political Terror*. New York: Basic Books.

Karatzias, Thanos, and Alytia A. Levendosky. 2019. Introduction to the Special Section on Complex Posttraumatic Stress Disorder (CPTSD): The Evolution of a Disorder. *Journal of Traumatic Stress* 32: 817–821. https://doi.org/10.1002/jts.22476.

Kezelman, Cathy, and Pam Stavropolous. 2019. *Practice Guidelines for Clinical Treatment of Complex Trauma*. Sydney: Blue Knot Foundation.

Kezelman, Cathy, and Pam Stavropolous. 2020. *Organisational Guidelines for Trauma-Informed Service Delivery*. Sydney: Blue Knot Foundation.

Lamb, Sharon. 1999. Constructing the Victim. Popular Images and Lasting Labels. In *New Versions of Victims. Feminists Struggle With the Concept*, ed. S. Lamb, 108–138. New York: New York University Press.

Levett, Ann. 2003. Problems of Cultural Imperialism in the Study of Child Sexual Abuse. In *New Feminist Stories of Child Sexual Abuse. Sexual Scripts and Dangerous Dialogues*, eds. P. Leavey and S. Warner, 52–76. London: Routledge.

Loney-Howes, Rachel. 2020. *Anti-Rape Activism: Exploring the Politics of the Personal in the Age of Digital Media*. Bingley: Emerald Publishing Limited.

Mardorossian, Carine M. 2002. Towards a New Feminist Theory of Rape. *Signs* 27: 743–775.

Marecek, Jeanne. 1999. Trauma Talk in Feminist Clinical Practice. In *New Versions of Victims. Feminist Struggle With the Concept,* ed. S. Lamb, 158–182. New York: New York University Press.

Mason, Gail. 2002. *The Spectacle of Violence: Homophobia, Gender, and Knowledge*. London: Routledge.

Müller, Ruth, and Martha Kenney. 2021. A Science of Hope? Tracing Emergent Entanglements Between the Biology of Early Life Adversity, Trauma-informed Care, and Restorative Justice. *Science, Technology, & Human Values* 46: 1230–1260. https://doi.org/10.1177/0162243920974095.

Health, New South Wales. 2020. *Responding to Sexual Assault (Child and Adult) Policies and Procedures*. Sydney: New South Wales Government.

O'Dell, Lindsey. 2003. The 'Harm' Story in Childhood Sexual Abuse: Contested Understandings, Disputed Knowledges. In *New Feminist Stories of Child Sexual Abuse. Sexual Scripts and Dangerous Dialogues,* eds. P. Leavey and S. Warner, 131–147. London: Routledge.

Pai, Anushka, Alina M. Suris, and Carol S. North. 2017. Posttraumatic Stress Disorder in the DSM-5: Controversy, Change, and Conceptual Considerations. *Behavioral Sciences* 7: 1–7.

Pickersgill, Martyn. 2018. The Value of the Imagined Biological in Policy and Society: Somaticizing and Economizing British Subject(ivitie)s. In *Handbook of Genomics, Health and Society,* eds S. Gibbon, B. Prainsack, S. Hilgartner and J. Lamoreaux, 99–107. New York: Routledge.

Rose, Nikolas, and Joelle M. Abi-Rached. 2013. *Neuro: The New Brain Sciences and the Management of the Mind*. Princeton, NJ: Princeton University Press.

Ruck, Nora, Vera Luckgei, Barbara Rothmüller, Nina Franke, and Emelie Rack. 2022. Psychologization In and Through the Women's Movement: A Transnational History of the Psychologization of Consciousness-raising in the German-speaking Countries and the United States. *Journal of the History of the Behavioral Sciences* 58: 269–290. https://doi.org/10.1002/jhbs.22187.

Stark, Eloise, Christine Parsons, Tim Van Hartevelt, Marine Charquero-Ballester, Hugh McManners, Anke Ehlers, Alan Stein, and Morten Kringelbach. 2015. Post-Traumatic Stress Influences the Brain Even in the Absence of Symptoms: A Systematic, Quantitative Meta-Analysis of Neuroimaging Studies. *Neuroscience and Behavioural Reviews* 56: 207–221.

Stark, Evan. 2007. *Coercive Control: How Men Entrap Women in Personal Life.* Oxford: Oxford University Press.

van der Kolk, Bessel. 2000. Posttraumatic Stress Disorder and the Nature of Trauma. *Dialogues in Clinical Neuroscience* 22: 7–22.

van der Kolk, Bessel. 2004. Psychobiology of Posttraumatic Stress Disorder. In *Textbook of Biological Psychiatry*, ed. J. Panksepp, 319–388. Hoboken, NJ: John Wiley & Sons.

van der Kolk, Bessel. 2015. *The Body Keeps the Score: Brain, Mind, and Body in the Healing of Trauma*. New York: Penguin Books.

Whittier, Nancy. 2009. *The Politics of Child Sexual Abuse. Emotions, Social Movements and the State*. Oxford: Oxford University Press.

Wilkin, Leslie, and Susan Hillock. 2014. Enhancing MSW Students' Efficacy in Working With Trauma, Violence, and Oppression: An Integrated Feminist-Trauma Framework for Social Work Education. *Feminist Teacher* 24: 184–206.

Young, Allan. 1995. *The Harmony of Illusions: The Invention of Post Traumatic Stress Disorder*. Princeton, NJ: Princeton University Press.

# Precarious Psy Expertise to Prevent Gender-Based Violence: The Case of Quebec

*Stéphanie Pache*

## 1 Introduction

In North America, most of the institutional policies developed to combat gender violence have concerned the aftermath of violence, predominantly within the justice sphere. They have led to better forensic care for the victims recognised as such, as well as financial support for organisations supporting victims (e.g. Delage 2017; Bruckert and Law 2018).[1] To a lesser extent, perpetrators of domestic violence have benefited from psycho-educational programs aimed at preventing recidivism, most often in conjunction with probation and prison services. These elements have been the subject of sociological and feminist research (e.g. Schneider 2002; Bevacqua 2008; Johnson 2012; Harper and Gover 2019; Gruber 2021; Douglas et al. 2024). The research on which this chapter is based focuses on a more ambitious initiative: rather than minimising the effects

[1] Several scholars emphasise how the recognition process mostly affects women with the means to navigate the legal system, including economic resources, but even more importantly respectability, which is not easily granted to non-white, non-straight women.

S. Pache (✉)
Université du Québec À Montréal, Montréal, QC, Canada
e-mail: pache.stephanie@uqam.ca



R. E. Keyse et al. (eds.), *Sexual Violence in Medicine and Psychiatry*, Genders and Sexualities in History,
https://doi.org/10.1007/978-3-032-10800-5_3

of violence by taking better care of victims and perpetrators, the aim is to prevent people from becoming victims and perpetrators in the first place. To this end, researchers, educators, social workers, and psychologists have created educational programs, inspired by psychological approaches and generally designed to be delivered in schools, universities or workplaces, to prevent the occurrence of sexist and sexual violence by spreading various communication techniques and sociological and psychological knowledge.

The scope of these programs is varied and their expressed target as multiform as gender violence: promoting healthy relationships or gender equality; constituting an education on consent; or presented more explicitly as sexual violence prevention and discussing sexual practices. In this aspect, they are the direct product of feminist problematisation of violence against women as a patriarchal strategy and feature. Their history and contemporary institutionalisation reflect this issue. In accordance with the feminist conception of gender violence as a continuum (Kelly 1987), I use here the analytical category of gender-based/gender violence to include diverse forms of violence. More concrete examples might however be limited to specific categories of violence, such as sexual violence or domestic violence.

This chapter takes as its case study a particular prevention project in Quebec, but also draws upon the broader North American context, examining the research supporting such programs and the grey literature produced by the non-profit, public, and private organisations that implement them.[2] Through reference to this grey literature, interviews conducted with workers and co-ordinators of prevention programs in Quebec, and documents such as program activity and evaluation reports, I analyse here the way in which violence prevention is conceived and organised by these organisations.

This chapter considers successively two forces at work in the development of these programs and the social and scientific construction of an expertise on gender violence prevention: psychological sciences and feminist movements. I discuss more specifically their imbrication in the case of

[2] I want to thank the two research assistants who helped me collect data for the Québec part of the research: Sarah Chaouch, who assisted me in organising and conducting four interviews with actors in the field of violence prevention, as much as in collecting data on the field; and Pascale Bilodeau, who conducted an ethnography of a conference on gender violence.

prevention programs in Quebec. This study shows, on one hand, a partial institutionalisation through the development of professional and scientific expertise, visible in particular in the number of resources produced for different audiences (for example, young people, parents, teachers, and the general public), programs offered to schools, and training provided to community and social service workers; on the other hand, we observe the singular precariousness of these intervention programs and the people who implement them.

## 2 The Making of Violence as a Preventable Behavioural Health Issue

### *2.1 Violence as Harm*

The notion that violence can and should be prevented through education and with behavioural techniques has a history. The emergence of the conception of violence as harm is one of the conditions that allows violence to become a public health issue and, consequently, to borrow medicalised language: epidemics, prevention, or the idea that violence can be 'eradicated'. But this view on violence, especially on interpersonal violence, is the product of social-historical processes that affected not only our ideas about violence but also how violence is framed as a social issue. In previous work I have retraced the different ways in which, over the last two centuries, interpersonal violence has been conceived as a public issue (Pache 2020). Interestingly, the shift to an almost exclusive focus on the harm of violence can be linked, though not exclusively, with political movements in the postwar period and the reframing of oppression as violence (Pache 2015, 2021). Mobilising a rhetoric of repression and liberation, power was then perceived mostly as a constraint over oppressed individuals and groups—and this constraint was equated with violence (Staub 2011). For their part, feminist movements emphasised the personal experience of oppression and denounced violence against women as inscribed in the patriarchal system (Kelly 1987). Their politicisation of intimate and sexual violence constructed it as the social issue that it is still today by making individual violent behaviours against women a feature of a collective dynamic of power, that is, patriarchy.

The association of violence with oppression seems to have fostered a view of any manifestation of oppression as violence and all violence as oppression. Violence is however not a concept with a stable definition, neither legally nor politically. The social construction of violence as a category has become particularly obvious with the expansion of behaviours that are qualified as violence nowadays: sometimes through political claims such as the criminalisation of rape in marriage in the 1980s or the implementation of policies against sexual harassment in the workplace, and sometimes through expert knowledge and professional practices, such as the expanding definition of bullying (Haslam 2016). But this expansion is made possible by the specific contemporary perspective on violence as harm, a process well supported by another social actor: psychology.

## 2.2 *Violence as an Object of Psychological Expertise*

As Herman (1995) showed, psychology assisted many social projects during the twentieth century in the United States. Mobilised to fight fascism, poverty, and racism, its expertise has been widely solicited, offered and endorsed by public actors. In modern liberal democracies, psy sciences—psychology, psychiatry, and psychoanalysis—seem to deliver a rational set of tools to 'improve' individual and collective behaviours, as much as productive theories to generate meaning from seemingly incomprehensible situations. However, as Herman points out, these 'policy-oriented' experts, like their clinical colleagues, are trained in the same mould and adopt a perspective conditioned by their training in the analysis of individual psychopathology, leading them to comprehend social problems and public policies on the same terms:

> One important result would be to blur the line between the individual and the collective, the personal and the social, and to create the potential for camouflaging clear political purposes as neutral methods of scientific discovery or therapeutic treatment. (Herman 1995: 22)

When social movements took a personal turn in postwar America, psychological expertise was so widely accepted that it served both these movements and their critics. Psychological analyses were published to explain civil rights activism or feminism, but activists also borrowed the language of madness and the legitimacy to assess rationality in order to denounce many oppressions and defend the idea that madness was a rational reaction to an irrational and oppressive world (Staub 2011). The relationship between the psy sciences and many social movements of this period, including feminist movements, was an ambivalent one. On one hand, feminists compellingly criticised the normative and conservative aspects of psychiatry, psychoanalysis, and psychology, and the role that these disciplines played in alliance with other oppressive institutions (e.g. the state, justice, medicine). On the other hand, they used their theories and practices to foster political approaches emphasising personal and interpersonal change to transform society more broadly. Activists also used psy expertise to demonstrate the damage done to oppressed individuals and to make this damage measurable.

Violence, and especially sexual violence and violence against women, did not escape this ambivalent examination by psy scientists. To underline the historical and contingent dimensions of our current views on gender violence, I review some of the ways psychological and behavioural sciences have looked at violence against women. I consider them in their social and scientific history, but this contextualisation should not be understood as a perfect chronology, nor a progression, since all these approaches co-exist and even combine to this day in one form or another, in the scientific field and society in general. Based mostly on a review of historical studies on violence (Pleck 1987; Gordon 2002; Peterson del Mar 2011; Bevacqua 2000; Freedman 2013; Akhtar 2017; Rutherford 2017b; Caplan 1985; Walker 2009; Cavalin 2016; Merry 2016; Delage 2017; Nicolson 2019), I propose to organise these perspectives according to their etiological centrality, which could also be defined as who is held responsible for violence from a primarily moral point of view, though it is also often linked to a legal dimension. Subsequently, four perspectives can be identified: (a) *aggressor-centred*, which focuses on the study of the aggressor and the factors that render a person aggressive; (b) *victim-centred*, with attention to how someone becomes a victim of violence; (c) *interpersonal*, emphasising the interpersonal dynamics of violence and the idea of conflict; and (d) *violence-focused*, which analyses the violent event itself, often around the notion of trauma.

### 2.2.1 *Aggressor-centred*

The first perspective, which can be designated as aggressor-centred, is in line with an ideal of progress. With the 'process of civilisation' (Elias 1973), Western societies seemingly developed intolerance towards interpersonal violence. The latter is seen as a loss of individual control, self-control itself being a new value that gradually became hegemonic over the course of the nineteenth century, which many authors (e.g. Weber 2017) link to the process of industrialisation and the birth of the bourgeoisie, effectively supported by Protestant values. Since the nineteenth century, several social reform movements—such as mental hygiene, social purity, and temperance movements—have framed violence as a sign of moral degeneration (Gordon 2002). The aggressor-centred perspective does not usually differentiate between categories of violence. It is concerned with aggression, almost exclusively considered to be masculine and linked with alcohol consumption and poverty.

What might seem like a view from the past is however still discernible in contemporary studies on aggression that pursue the same lines of investigation for a biological explanation of violent behaviours, a view also popular in the public (Weidman 2021). In addition, violence against women is not seen by everyone as problematic, and male violence is often linked to supposed biological differences between the sexes. In particular, the hypothesis that testosterone explains male aggression and posits this as necessary for the evolution of the species, is still current despite the lack of data justifying it and numerous studies and analyses contesting it (Longino 2013). It is against this first and hegemonic perspective on violence as aggression and aggressor-centred that other studies and views on violence were developed, including those that support violence prevention (e.g. Albee 1996).

### 2.2.2 *Victim-centred*

In early twentieth century psy sciences, interpersonal violence was mainly examined by criminologists and psychologists who were confronted with criminal cases. In the United States of America, much research and legislation dealing with psychopathy was influenced by concerns over sexual violence perpetrated by strangers (e.g. Freedman 2006, 121–139). This work reinforced the idea that violence and abuse in the private sphere were relatively rare. Psychoanalysis, as a newly established approach to the human mind, offered psy experts a satisfactory framework for understanding violent behaviours that were relabelled as 'perversions' and 'personality disorders' under this lens. These psychoanalytical interpretations became hegemonic enough to be taken up by criminologists and, by the 1950s, spread to the point where rape victims were commonly accused of 'secretly having asked for it' (Akhtar 2017). In particular, the idea of female masochism was mobilised to explain the victimisation of women, who were understood to have an unconscious desire to become victims. Through this lens, both sexual and domestic violence victims were portrayed as unconsciously willing. Unsurprisingly, the paternalism of psychoanalysis and the use of masochism as an explanation that dismissed the responsibility of the perpetrator of violence, became the target of considerable feminist criticisms (Caplan 1985; Buhle 1998). However, psychoanalysis also paved the way for psychological explanations of violent behaviour and for a shift towards the study of the subjective experience of violence. It supported theories postulating a rational use of violence, even if the rationality may be unconscious, and as such, this perspective challenged the notion that violence is the product of a lack of self-control. By considering the effects of experience and of its subjective interpretation, psychodynamic approaches also offered conceptual tools for understanding the impact of violence, including the controversial and reinterpreted notion of traumatic neurosis (Leys 2000), but also the concept of microaggression (Pierce 1970; Pache 2025).

### 2.2.3 *Interpersonal*

The immediate post-war period (1945–1960) put the family at the centre of government concerns, as the matrix of citizens and therefore a focus for action to prevent fascism, as much as social and racial inequalities.[3] Family therapy was formed in this context, a clinical practice which stemmed from psychoanalysis but also drew inspiration from cybernetics, a theory of communication focused on chains of signals and feedback. Family therapists observed what they called 'pathological family interactions' with the aim of changing communication dynamics and preventing psychiatric illnesses (e.g. schizophrenia), but also social issues, such as racism or youth delinquency (Weinstein 2013). In its early form, family therapy rarely addressed the problem of intra-family violence, drawing much criticism from later feminist therapists (e.g. Goodrich 1991). However, its relevance lies in the way family therapists reframed interpersonal violence as a conflict caused by communication issues, which invisibilised, denied, or sometimes justified power relations. In this conception, responsibility for violence is therefore *inter-personal*, i.e. in between individuals, so no single individual is to blame. Its emphasis is on the capacity—and thus to some extent the responsibility—of everyone involved in the system

[3] The fight against these inequalities was also part of the action plan to promote democracy, as inequalities were seen as a breeding ground for anti-democratic endencies, which were attributed both to fascist and communist ideology in the postwar United States.

to change the dynamics. This conception invisibilises power differentials and their roots in social institutions such as family and patriarchy. This interpersonal perspective removes violence from its broader social and political dimensions, but remains popular in some institutions focused on family and its preservation, as the Québec context will show. Cybernetic ideas about communication and systems theory stressing the benefits of self-regulation spread in the 1970s to the point that this 'culture of feedback' (Belgrad 2019) pervaded cultural representations of the techniques that can instigate change. Infused by hopeful belief in the capacity of humans to reflect and 'self-regulate' through feedback loops, countercultural initiatives renewed the conceptualisation of social responsibility by placing intersubjectivity at the centre of an 'ecological ethic' (Belgrad 2019). Outside family therapy, I suggest that this approach permeates views on prevention of violence, in particular the emphasis on communication, while the role of social hierarchies is rarely addressed explicitly in prevention programs against interpersonal violence.

#### *2.2.4 Violence-focused*

Focused on the violent event itself, the last perspective on violence conceptualises the phenomenon through its consequences: trauma and the post-traumatic stress disorder (PTSD). Historically related to the recognition of disabilities engendered by work accidents and wars, the debate on traumatic neurosis evolved radically in the second half of the twentieth century (Leys 2000). In this period, influenced by emerging narratives published by concentration camp survivors, trauma was recognised as an effect of violence for the first time. However, this perspective was not fully institutionalised in American psychiatry until the 1970s, under pressure from Vietnam War veterans and their psychiatrists. This led to the acceptance of the view that some traumatic events alone can explain psychological distress and symptoms, moving away from the previous view underlining predispositions of affected individuals (Fassin and Rechtman 2007). The PTSD category was included in the 1980 third revision of the *Diagnostic and Statistical Manual of Mental Disorders* (*DSM*), with feminist support (Young 1995). This recognition of the 'victim condition' (Fassin and Rechtman 2007) posited that violence has universal effects, that any individual could present the same symptoms when facing a traumatic event. This depathologising effort reinscribed the psychological approach of violence and the framing of trauma as a health issue. Since, in this framing, post-traumatic effects are standardised, and anyone can be traumatised, this approach is compatible with the public health agenda and efforts to prevent violence. In this framework, trauma is the key concept that marks violence as harm and formalises this harm as *primarily* psychological. In this perspective, violence *can* indeed cause physical trauma, but *at least* a psychological one, which is then the necessary but sufficient criterion to testify to the experience of violence. Once the harm caused to (mental) health by interpersonal violence has been established, prevention can appear as a legitimate course of action. However, other social dynamics were necessary to put violence prevention on the public agenda.

## 3 Feminism, Gender-Based Violence and Psychology

The fight against sexist violence was and still is a defining cause for feminist movements. Therefore, it does not come as a surprise that committed feminist activists and practitioners were concerned by this issue since the first anti-violence feminist actions in the 1970s. Gender-based violence continues to be an object of research and treatment, and thus a field of professional development, both in academia and in clinical practice. Feminist psychologists have designed both a feminist psychology and a feminist therapy (Pache 2015, 2016). Actors against gender-based violence have also developed a specific scientific expertise, and this new knowledge has helped them publicise the problem and legitimise public programs (e.g., Rutherford 2017b). However, the project of feminist researchers and practitioners in the field of gender violence blurs the boundaries between political commitment and the production of scientific knowledge. In this respect, it is in line with the feminist epistemologies of science developed since 1970 (Puig de la Bellacasa 2012). This raises key questions: how can the research methods of public health and behavioural sciences fit in with a feminist politics of knowledge? Can it be better described as an 'epistemological mosaic', a configuration that would be designed by an assemblage of different epistemologies? But then, might the possible inconsistencies weaken both fields, political and scientific?

This point has very practical implications, particularly for the study and management of violence. The question of defining what constitutes violence, and of locating the threshold of violence that justifies intervention or sanction, is eminently problematic, as illustrated by the difficulty victims have in making themselves heard and believed rather than having their experiences delegitimised or downplayed (Alcoff 2018). It is thus crucial to understand what forms of expertise are considered legitimate in the documentation, assessment, and analysis of the experience of violence, as well as how these forms of expertise are used to justify different types of intervention (e.g. educational, social, therapeutic, or judicial). The standardisation of the experience of violence within psychological categories also potentially fails to account for the diversity of subjective experiences and to offer appropriate support to victims. Because of the power relations at the heart of the production of these categories, standardised categories risk reproducing social hierarchies (i.e. race, age and class).

To examine the programs developed in Quebec, this chapter analyses the institutionalisation of prevention practices against violence with these issues in mind. It considers the kind of psychological expertise that is mobilised to legitimate prevention programs, as much as what this expertise is 'doing' to these programs. But after presenting the role of psychology and its ambivalent relationship with feminism, it is necessary to understand the role of the national and provincial political history and the contemporary situation with regard to the politics of violence against women.

## 4 Gender-Based Violence as a Public Issue

### *4.1 Canada*

Canada is often presented as a country with progressive policies regarding health and gender-based violence, and even as a model for progressive social policies. In many cases, Canadian actions and policies seem to be a continuation, almost an extension, of those in the United States, but appear to be implemented with greater ease (Weldon 2002). In the case of violence against women, we can observe similar strategies in both countries: documenting violence with large-scale population surveys; using the same (American) typologies of violence (e.g. Johnson 2008); and reforming victim support services and legal procedures. More recently, scholars have started to question the 'niceness' associated with Canada, especially through an intersectional lens (Bruckert and Law 2018) and to highlight tensions between the feminist approach to gender-based violence and its contemporary institutionalisation in a context of right-wing federal and provincial governments, which employ a capitalist and nationalist strategy in which anti-violence work is funded on a project basis, and funding is routinely cut (Brodie 2008; Flynn et al. 2018).

As in most national contexts where the issue of gender-based violence has been raised as such, feminist movements were essential in raising public awareness on the topic. With the establishment of shelters for women and services for rape victims from the early 1970s, feminist activists and professionals were at the forefront of the battle. The Canadian state is praised for putting violence against women on its agenda as early as 1974 (Lundy 2022: 59) and for taking action, first funding research and services such as crisis centres and shelters, and then by introducing legal reforms to encourage reporting and prosecuting of rape and domestic violence (Weldon 2002).

Following the analysis of Weldon (2002), Lundy (2022) explains this early action in the context of a strong Canadian women's movement and a 'responsive government'. She notes how the government engaged 'women's organisations in a 'consult and study' process and provid[ed] minimal funding to a network of women's organisations while choosing to emphasise legal and policy changes' (Lundy 2022: 59). These reforms mostly affected the judicial system. Several authors consider this federal strategy with ambivalence. Lundy (2022) notices how the critique of Sandra Preston (1999) fits in with Weldon's (2002):

> Preston sees the results of such an approach as both laudable and problematic as each group of women steered certain aspects of the violence against women agenda, leaving the state with significant room to create a system that meets state needs, at times to the detriment of women living in or leaving violent relationships. (Lundy 2022: 60)

State funding for women's groups and networks has diminished across the years, leading to the disappearance of some national organisations as early as the 1990s. The attack by Marc Lépine, who killed fourteen women on December 6, 1989, at the École Polytechnique in Montreal, provoked increased public awareness and a visible response from the federal government. But this response was limited to convening experts to discuss gendered violence and reporting about it; it did not prompt the government to fund a federal response against gender-based violence. Lundy (2022) cites Weldon's (2002) comparative analysis, and her conclusion that 'the responsiveness of a state does not automatically imply effectiveness of the actions', in her critique of the Canadian example, where, while the 'government launched initiatives to study the problem and engage in consultation with women's groups, decisions were also made to drastically reduce funding to the very groups that provide frontline support and services to women' (Lundy 2022, 61).

In 2017, the Federal Government announced a new initiative 'It's Time: Canada's Strategy to Prevent and Address Gender-Based Violence' (Gouvernement du Canada 2017). The federal program had a budget of $850 million for the 2017–2026 period, including $40 million provided as emergency funding for shelters during the Covid-19 pandemic. The plan supported research, awareness initiatives, and services for victims. This most recent federal strategy expanded the old procedures to diverse publics: quantifying and characterising the violence experienced by minorities (First Nations, LGBTQ*, immigrant persons, etc.), by other means (technologies, social media), and at different ages (bullying in school, teen dating violence, etc.); multiplying communication tools (webinars, toolkits, leaflet, etc.,); supporting permanently underfunded services (shelters, victim support services, etc.); and increasing the criminalisation of intimate partner and sexual violence.

### 4.2 *Quebec*

The same dynamics in public actions and funding are at work in the province of Quebec. Nevertheless, in 1995, Quebec's first plan to combat violence against women established violence as the product of power relations and gender-based social relations, a definition that has been adopted in subsequent plans despite controversy and attempts to change it to include a more behavioural and legal definition of intimate partner violence. The Quebec network of shelters and services for victims still identify strongly with feminism, and the social workers and other professionals working in the field of domestic and sexual violence deplore the defunding or chronic underfunding of their organisations.

In line with the rest of Canada and elsewhere in the world, many Quebec feminist professionals and scholars working with women victims of violence contend that (1) they are witnessing a more or less successful attempt to depoliticise gender-based violence; (2) this depoliticisation consists in invisibilising the collective dynamics of gender equality, and conceptualising violence as an individual behaviour; (3) this conceptualisation can be seen in psychologisation processes, whether through the terminology used or the type of actions proposed, such as therapy or legal procedures (e.g. Flynn et al. 2022). Family therapy, which, as discussed earlier, often approaches violence as a communication problem, is well established in Quebec. However, it might be too rushed to label systemic therapists as agents of masculinism (even if some of them are such agents) without examining how their power of influence and the legitimacy attributed to their positions are rooted in the same social, professional, and scientific institutions that support feminist psychologists' expertise: the many institutions—such as universities, states, and the media—that grant power and legitimacy to such expertise. So, rather than opposing a feminist definition to a psychological approach to violence, it might be useful to examine how feminists also use psychologists and psychology. Likewise, the tension between the Quebec government's feminist definition of gender violence and a capitalist management of its budget cannot be treated separately from the politics of knowledge involved in this debate. Therefore, to a large part, Quebec is just another part of North America, characterised by underfunded public services and the need to build private-public partnerships, which in the violence sector means that community organisations are proactively fundraising through foundations, as well as perpetually submitting 'new' projects to the State to maintain their activities.

Quebec is not exempt from the psychological culture found in most Western countries, together with the touch of scientistic belief prevalent in North American approaches to public issues. In this context, psychological expertise is crucial for the implementation of new policies (Herman 1995), as is the quantification of the problem and measurement of the efficacy of policies (Merry 2016). The technocratic rationalisation of politics through data production is enhanced by psychological research and reports, as illustrated by the constant multiplication of victimisation surveys trying to measure the occurrence of the experience of violence to support policies against gender-based violence (Merry 2016). Numbers give the appearance of objectivity and seem to support rational choice and psychological methods that can be defended as a necessary scientific social engineering (e.g. Rutherford 2017a). In the case of gender-based violence, numbers are repeatedly contested, as is, relatedly, its definition. The science of violence, especially gender-based violence, remains very political, which explains feminist scholars' involvement in support of public actions in this technocratic and capitalist environment. Of course, as I have previously suggested (Pache 2015, 2019), it is expected that feminist psychologists would contribute to feminist claims, such as the fight against gender violence. But the more relevant question to ask is why feminist activists and social workers, while complaining about the psychologisation of violence, rely on psychology and its expertise to support their action?[4]

## 5 Prevention Programs in Quebec

In this cultural context, prevention is welcomed by feminists as collective action through education. This support is mirrored by the main stakeholders of the domestic violence sector. However, educational programs are harder to fund and implement: they require collaboration with schools, therefore also necessitating cooperation between several government ministries; they are difficult to standardise and their effectiveness, more diffuse, is also more difficult to implement and assess formally; and it is not straightforward to define who are the experts in such prevention or how to train professionals to undertake this task.

Neither in Canada nor in Quebec is the prevention of gender violence covered by legislation that would make it a mandatory school activity. As a result, several initiatives have developed in parallel, sometimes reinforcing each other, sometimes going their separate ways. The conducted empirical study showed the singular precariousness of these intervention programs and the people who implement them, linked as much to financial issues as to political ones. These conditions were obvious from the outset of the research, manifesting in both the difficulty of access to the field and the lack of availability of key actors, as quite a few of them had moved on to other fields of work when funding for particular prevention projects ceased.

In Quebec, two dynamics are driving the campaign for a systematic implementation of standardised prevention programs against sexual violence. The first emerged in 2010 from the network of the Quebec Coalition of Sexual Assault Help Centers (its French acronym being RQCALACS) (Bergeron et al. 2014). Concerned about the long-term viability of their prevention initiatives, the 23 Quebec Sexual Assault Help Centers wanted to pool their resources and set up a joint program.

[4] Psychology is only the second most mobilised expertise in this field, the first being the one offered by feminist legal scholars, which, despite indisputable links, is not discussed in this chapter. For a discussion of how law and psy expertise are intertwined in the context of sexual violence, see Marriner (2012).

They partnered with Manon Bergeron, a professor in the Department of Sexology at Université du Québec à Montréal (UQAM), to collect data about their practices and define what a common prevention program should look like. The consultation allowed them to identify a series of themes for a program (Bergeron et al. 2014). In 2015, with additional funding and partners, including Bergeron's colleague, Martine Hébert—a psychologist specialised in youth relationships, sexual violence and trauma—the same team proposed a prevention program called *Empreinte* (imprint), which comprised a 6-session program for secondary school students (i.e. 12–15 years old), training for teachers, and materials (short videos) for parents (Bergeron et al. 2018). In 2019, the *Étincelles/SPARX* program, led by Martine Hébert and supported by the Public Health Agency of Canada, was launched. This program 'aims to promote positive intimate and romantic relationships and prevent dating violence among high school youth' (Étincelles/SPARX n.d.). Beside these two programs, other programs and actions are created and conducted in schools by community organisations mandated directly by the schools.

The second force pushing for a legal framework to support funding and mandatory implementation of prevention activities against sexual violence comes from a youth movement supported by community organisers. In 2018, the collective *La voix des jeunes compte* ('the voice of youth counts') was founded in Montreal, comprised of girls and women aged between 11 and 21, who denounced the sexual violence they had experienced or observed. The initiative emerged from the activities of the community centre *La Maison d'Haïti* and its program *Juste pour elles* ('only for them'), which offers formal and informal activities for girls in women-and-girls-only spaces (La Maison d'Haïti n.d.). The *La voix de jeunes compte* collective is supported by a coalition of organisations defending Quebec's adoption of a legal framework to fund and implement prevention programs in every school, comparable to an anti-bullying policy that was adopted previously. This coalition calls itself *Mouvement pour des écoles sans violences sexuelles* (MESVS), which translates into English as 'movement for schools without sexual violence'. The movement provides logistical support to the collective, particularly in terms of event organisation and communication. This coalition claims more explicitly to be part of the #MeToo campaign and mobilises politicians and political institutions to support legal changes. Sharing actors and projects, these two vectors of change mobilise similar strategies to legitimise the need of prevention programs. For example, the organisation *Prévention-CDN-NDG*,[5] which is a member of MESVS, also conducted a project to assess the needs for sexual harassment prevention in schools (Prévention CDN-NDG 2019). This initiative was supposed to be run in three parts: (1) consultation and recommendations; (2) creation of tools; (3) implementation. However, only the first part was conducted, because of staff and funding shortages.

## 6 The Politics of Psycho Mumbo Jumbo

This study borrows questions and methods of feminist science studies by subjecting the data collected from actors in the field of violence prevention to a critical analysis of the construction of a feminist expertise on gender violence prevention in Quebec. It examined the discourses and techniques involved in the scientific and institutional construction of the prevention practices. These violence prevention programs can be seen as the deployment of feminist and psychological expertise against gender-based violence, this expertise itself being the product of the conflict of expertise between the two fields. This approach serves to identify the modalities of elaboration, implementation and expected effects of the violence prevention project. It exposes this project as composed by a network of actors with diverse expertise and sometimes convergent objectives.

Political and economic dynamics shed light on the use of experts and their psychological expertise in this contemporary context. In many national contexts, public funding is subject to specific evaluations of need and efficacy. Such funding regimes render the funded programs precarious, a fact that is also reinforced by the contingency of shifting political forces. The multiplication of partnerships with academic researchers results in the proliferation of rather comparable reports recommending similar policies, based on analogous methods and identical literature. If the strategic dimensions of the enterprise are understandable, the almost systematic partnership with researchers from psychology or associated disciplines such as sexology or social work also betrays the legitimacy granted to these approaches and their methods.

[5] Côtes des neiges (CDN) and Notre-Dame-de-Grâce (NDG) are two neighborhoods of Montreal composing the city district of Côte-des-Neiges–Notre-Dame-de-Grâce.

Beyond their similarities, the reports analysed show how the proposed prevention programs consist of psycho-educational workshops and materials meant to foster behavioural change. If the expressed goal is preventing violence, especially sexual violence, the researchers mostly propose to assess the efficacy of the programs through psychological measures, such as the sense of self-efficacy, self-esteem, leadership capacity, and 'attitude' towards sexual violence, in addition to acquired knowledge (Fernet et al. 2022). In their review of prevention programs with peer mentors, Fernet et al. (2022) noted that only one program had measured the impact on the incidence of sexual violence.

This research seeks to understand what kinds of knowledge and expertise are mobilised by professionals in violence prevention and to extend our questioning of the role of psychology in public action against gender violence in North America (Pache 2021). The case of prevention programs shows the relevance of an analysis that focuses less on the conflict between fields of action (political struggle, public action, psychology, or education) and more on how these modes of action and their own logics hybridise to achieve shared, or rather negotiated, objectives. When, for example, violence prevention becomes the 'promotion of healthy relationships', with the explicit aim of not being put off by a 'negative' subject and of including everyone—meaning girls and boys—in prevention activities with a 'positive' objective, this is one such negotiation.

As I have shown by reviewing psychological conceptions of interpersonal violence, violent behaviour is the subject of psychological analyses that are: (1) long-standing, which makes it difficult to speak of the psychologisation of violence, including gender-based violence, as recent[6]; and (2) contradictory, reflecting the less homogeneous nature of the field and the necessarily political dimension that scientific debates assume on this topic. What does the recourse to psychological expertise by the actors in the field of violence mean, when at the same time they criticise the depoliticisation of gender-based violence through its psychologisation? Ultimately, we can see here that they draw a distinction between the

[6] As noted by others, such as Sunny Marriner, who has worked for decades with victims of sexual assault in Ottawa, wrote in a text 'questioning "expert" knowledges' that 'it is plain that sexual violence is *still* directly linked with "mental health issues", *despite* years of feminist work to establish that reacting to sexual violence is reasonable, not indicative of poor mental health.' (Marriner 2012: 429, my emphasis).

'feminist' psychology of their allies and the one threatening their services and their conception of gender violence. We can also recognise it as an alliance that mutualises and reinforces their reciprocal professional and scientific expertise. These research partnerships might not produce much knowledge, but they empower both sides of the partnership through the hybridisation of expertise, which contribute to legitimise researchers in the eyes of a capitalist state obsessed with 'applied' research, as much as to grant quasi-scientific quality to the professionals' expertise through quantification, standardised methods and measures of efficacy.

The first issue is that this strategy does not work politically to assure the political support and funding of prevention programs. Year after year, for more than 20 years, in Quebec and elsewhere in North America, we can draw a chronology of studies and reports showing the need for more funding in prevention. The idea that the only obstacle to effective gender-based violence prevention is a lack of funding is widely held among actors in the field of violence, feminist researchers and activists. However, these actions fit too perfectly with the technocratic nature of the contemporary capitalist state and academia.

The second and more critical issue relates to the question of expertise and its legitimacy. As Herman (1995) reminds us about other social reformers in psy disciplines, feminist psychologists are still psychologists trained in the same institutions and benefitting from the same privileges as other psychologists. They might use their social capital for the greater feminist good, but the feminist psychological or professional expertise replays social hierarchies that are problematic both for gender equality, especially in relation to its intersectional challenges, and for women in general, as much as for victims of violence. Yet, it remains to be discussed who would be the experts on preventing gender-based violence and if there should be any. The kind of large-scale social change that the 'eradication' of violence requires seems to be a matter for collective political action. Its framing as a behavioural change that can be enforced in school programs transforms the issue into a psychological one, and grants psychologists' expertise on the subject, even if this expertise is far from being scientifically or experientially grounded. The trust in feminist psychology can therefore be analysed as the restoration or the reinforcement of the power of expertise, although feminist movements have severely condemned experts—and especially psy experts—as undermining women's power and credibility. As we have seen, the psychological encoding of gender-based violence as a behavioural issue can take many forms, including some that are now supported by some feminists. Each one of them is embedded however in a system of norms that pretends to state truths that could be attested by experts, rather than defend values that can be argued politically and democratically. The warning of the historian of science Dominique Pestre resonates both with feminist critiques of expertise and with current claims of feminist expertise:

> beware of those who play the science card, who tell you that they speak in its name—and who often use one social characterisation to invalidate the other and add to the argument of authority. The will to do science is first and foremost an intention, need we remind you? (Pestre 2001: 181, my translation)

**Funding** This research was supported by Fonds de recherche du Québec—Société et culture (FRQSC), Grant Number 2022-NP-296180. The author declares no competing interests.

## References

Akhtar, Leena Mehreen. 2017. *From Masochists to Traumatized Victims: Psychiatry, Law, and the Feminist Anti-Rape Movement of the 1970s*. PhD diss., Harvard University.

Albee, George W. 1996. The Psychological Origins of the White Male Patriarchy. *Journal of Primary Prevention* 17: 75–97. https://doi.org/10.1007/BF02262739.

Alcoff, Linda. 2018. *Rape and Resistance: Understanding the Complexities of Sexual Violation*. Cambridge: Polity Press.

Belgrad, Daniel. 2019. *The Culture of Feedback: Ecological Thinking in Seventies America*. Chicago: The University of Chicago Press.

Bergeron, Manon, Annie Girard, and Regroupement québécois des CALACS. 2014. *Analyse des pratiques préventives des CALACS en matière d'agression à caractère sexuel dans les écoles secondaires du Québec: à la recherche de balises communes*. Montréal: Département de sexologie et Service aux collectivités, Université du Québec à Montréal.

Bergeron, Manon, Martine Hébert, Geneviève Brodeur, Anne-Julie Bouchard, Katherine Jodoin, Marily Julien, and Regroupement québécois des CALACS. 2018. *Rapport d'évaluation des effets du programme Empreinte - Agir ensemble contre les agressions à caractère sexuel*. Montréal: Université du Québec à Montréal.

Bevacqua, Maria. 2000. *Rape on the Public Agenda: Feminism and the Politics of Sexual Assault*. Boston: Northeastern University Press.

Bevacqua, Maria. 2008. Reconsidering Violence Against Women: Coalition Politics in the Antirape Movement. In *Feminist Coalitions: Historical Perspectives on Second-Wave Feminism in the United States*, ed. Stephanie Gilmore, 163–177. Urbana, IL: University of Illinois Press.

Brodie, Janine. 2008. We Are All Equal Now: Contemporary Gender Politics in Canada. *Feminist Theory* 9: 145–164. https://doi.org/10.1177/1464700108090408.

Bruckert, Chris, and Tuulia Law. 2018. *Women and Gendered Violence in Canada: An Intersectional Approach*. Toronto: University of Toronto Press.

Buhle, Mari Jo. 1998. *Feminism and its Discontents: A Century of Struggle With Psychoanalysis*. Cambridge, MA: Harvard University Press.

Caplan, Paula J. 1985. *The Myth of Women's Masochism*, 1st ed. New York: Dutton.

Cavalin, Catherine. 2016. *Objectivations savante et objet de politiques publiques: les violences interpersonnelles dans les habits neufs de la statistique et de la santé publique (France/Europe/États-Unis, 1995–2016)*. PhD diss., Sciences Po.

Delage, Pauline. 2017. *Violences conjugales: Du combat féministe à la cause publique*. Paris: SciencePo les presses.

Douglas, Heather, Kate Fitz-Gibbon. Heather, Leigh Goodmark, and Sandra Walklate, eds. 2024. *The Criminalization of Violence Against Women: Comparative Perspectives*. Oxford: Oxford University Press.

Elias, Norbert. 1973. *La civilisation des moeurs*. Paris: Calmann-Lévy.

Étincelles/SPARX. n.d. What Is Sparx? https://etincelles.uqam.ca/en/. Accessed on 9 September 2024.

Fassin, Didier, and Richard Rechtman. 2007. *L'empire du traumatisme. Enquête sur la condition de victime*. Paris: Flammarion.

Fernet, Mylène, Martine Hébert, Jacinthe Dion, Andréanne Fortin, Geneviève Brodeur, Camille Dupuis, and Myriam Day Asselin. 2022. Une Synthèse Des Programmes Ciblant L'entraide Par Les Pairs En Matière De Violence Dans Les Relations Amoureuses À L'adolescence. In *Pratiques et recherches féministes en matière de violence conjugale*, ed. Mylène Fernet, Carole Boulebsol, Marie- Cousineau, Chloé Deraiche, Catherine Flynn, Sylvie Genest, Estibaliz Jimenez, and Josiane Maheu, 111–126. Quebec: Presses de l'Université du Québec.

Flynn, Catherine, Pénélope. Couturier, Charlotte Gagnon, Josiane Maheu, Gaëlle. Fedida, Louise Lafortune, Manon Monastesse, and Marie Cousineau. 2018. Violence conjugale et intervention féministe au Québec – les défis d'une pratique subversive dans un contexte de politiques néolibérales. *Nouvelles Questions Feministes* 37: 47–63.

Flynn, Catherine, Josiane Maheu, Julie Godin, and Élie. Fortin-Otis. 2022. Les définitions théorique, politique et empirique de la violence conjugale lorsque la neutralité contribue à réaffirmer la domination masculine. In *Pratiques et recherches féministes en matière de violence conjugale*, ed. Carole Boulebsol, Marie- Cousineau, Chloé Deraiche, Mylène Fernet, Catherine Flynn, Sylvie Genest, Estibaliz Jimenez, and Josiane Maheu, 35–49. Quebec: Presses de l'Université du Québec.

Freedman, Estelle B. 2006. *Feminism, Sexuality, and Politics: Essays*. Chapel Hill, NC: University of North Carolina Press.

Freedman, Estelle B. 2013. *Redefining Rape: Sexual Violence in the Era of Suffrage and Segregation*. Cambridge, MA: Harvard University Press.

Goodrich, Thelma Jean, ed. 1991. *Women and Power: Perspectives for Family Therapy*. New York: W. W. Norton & Company.

Gordon, Linda. 2002. *Heroes of Their Own Lives: The Politics and History of Family Violence: Boston, 1880–1960*. Urbana: University of Illinois Press.

Gouvernement du Canada. 2017. *Il est temps: La Stratégie du Canada pour prévenir et contrer la violence fondée sur la sexe*. www.canada.ca/fr/femmes-egalite-genres/violence-fondee-sexe/strategie-contre-violence-fondee-sexe.html. Accessed on 9 September 2024.

Gruber, Aya. 2021. *The Feminist War on Crime: The Unexpected Role of Women's Liberation in Mass Incarceration*. Oakland, CA: University of California Press.

Harper, Shannon B., and Angela R. Gover. 2019. A Feminist Perspective on the Criminal Justice System Response to Domestic Violence. In *Handbook of Interpersonal Violence Across the Lifespan*, eds. Robert Geffner, Victor Vieth, Viola Vaughan-Eden, Alan Rosenbaum, L. Kevin Hamberger, and Jacquelyn White, 1–30. Cham: Springer International Publishing. https://doi.org/10.1007/978-3-319-62122-7_203-1.

Haslam, Nick. 2016. Concept Creep: Psychology's Expanding Concepts of Harm and Pathology. *Psychological Inquiry* 27: 1–17. https://doi.org/10.1080/1047840X.2016.1082418.

Herman, Ellen. 1995. *The Romance of American Psychology*. Berkeley: University of California Press.

Johnson, Holly. 2012. Limits of a Criminal Justice Response: Trends in Police and Court Processing of Sexual Assault. In *Sexual Assault in Canada*, ed. Elizabeth A. Sheehy, 613–634. Ottawa: University of Ottawa Press.

Johnson, Michael P. 2008. *A Typology of Domestic Violence: Intimate Terrorism, Violent Resistance, and Situational Couple Violence*. Boston: Northeastern University Press.

Kelly, Liz. 1987. The Continuum of Sexual Violence. In *Women, Violence and Social Control*, eds. Jalna Hanmer and Mary Maynard, 46–60. London: Palgrave Macmillan. https://doi.org/10.1007/978-1-349-18592-4_4.

La Maison d'Haïti. n.d. *Jeunesse: Juste pour Elles*. https://www.mhaiti.org/web/jeunesse-juste-pour-elles/. Accessed on 9 September 2024.

Leys, Ruth. 2000. *Trauma: A Genealogy*. Chicago, IL: University of Chicago Press.

Longino, Helen E. 2013. *Studying Human Behavior: How Scientists Investigate Aggression and Sexuality*. Chicago, IL: University of Chicago Press.

Lundy, Colleen. 2022. Violence Against Women: A Structural Perspective. In *Cruel But Not Unusual: Violence in Families in Canada*, ed. Ramona Alaggia and Cathy Vine, 43–74. Waterloo, Ontario: Wilfrid Laurier University Press.

Marriner, Sunny. 2012. Questioning "Expert" Knowledges. In *Sexual Assault in Canada*, ed. Elizabeth A. Sheehy, 409–450. Ottawa: University of Ottawa Press.

Merry, Sally Engle. 2016. *The Seductions of Quantification: Measuring Human Rights, Gender Violence, and Sex Trafficking*. Chicago: The University of Chicago Press.

Nicolson, Paula. 2019. *Domestic Violence and Psychology: Critical Perspectives on Intimate Partner Violence and Abuse*, 2nd ed. New York: Routledge.

Pache, Stéphanie. 2015. *Politiser la psychologie. Histoire d'une théorie féministe de la pratique psychothérapeutique (États-Unis, 1960–2015)*. PhD diss., Université de Lausanne.

Pache, Stéphanie. 2016. Entre science et politique: La question épistémologique dans l'histoire de la psychologie féministe. *Recherches Féministes* 29: 33–50. https://doi.org/10.7202/1036668ar.

Pache, Stéphanie. 2019. L'histoire féministe de la « psychologisation des violences ». *Cahiers du Genre* 66 (1): 51–70. https://doi.org/10.3917/cdge.066.0051.

Pache, Stéphanie. 2020. A History of Interpersonal Violence: Raising Public Concern. In *Handbook of Interpersonal Violence Across the Lifespan*, eds. Robert Geffner, Victor Vieth, Viola Vaughan-Eden, Alan Rosenbaum, L. Kevin Hamberger, and Jacquelyn White, 1–22. Cham: Springer International Publishing. https://doi.org/10.1007/978-3-319-62122-7_284-1.

Pache, Stéphanie. 2021. 'Healthy' Relationships: Feminism and the Psy Disciplines in the Political History of Sexual Violence in Contemporary America. In *Histories of Sexology*, eds. Alain Giami and Sharman Levinson, 61–79. Cham: Springer International Publishing. https://doi.org/10.1007/978-3-030-65813-7_4.

Pache, Stéphanie. 2022. Rendre sensible l'expérience de violence. La souffrance psychique dans les luttes contre les violences sexistes aux États-Unis, des années 1970 à #MeToo. In *Les violences sexistes après #MeToo*, eds. Catherine Cavalin, Jaércio Da Silva, Pauline Delage, Irène Despontin Lefèvre, Delphine Lacombe, and Bibia Pavard, 197–209. Paris: Presses des Mines.

Pache, Stéphanie. 2025. Chester Middlebrook Pierce and the Birth of Microaggression. *History of Psychology 28* (4): 298–311. https://doi.org/10.1037/hop0000287.

Pestre, Dominique. 2001. Études sociales des sciences, politique et retour sur soi. Éléments pour sortir d'un débat convenu. *Revue Du MAUSS* 17: 180–196. https://doi.org/10.3917/rdm.017.0180.

Peterson del Mar, David. 2011. *Beaten Down: A History of Interpersonal Violence in the West*. Seattle, WA: University of Washington Press.

Pierce, Chester M. 1970. Offensive Mechanisms. In *The Black Seventies*, ed. Floyd B. Barbour, 264–282. Boston: Porter Sargent.

Pleck, Elizabeth H. 1987. *Domestic Tyranny: The Making of Social Policy Against Family Violence from Colonial Times to the Present*. New York: Oxford University Press.

Preston, Sandra. 1999. The Glass Half Full: Responses to Woman Abuse by the Federal and Ontario Governments, 1980–1995. *Canadian Review of Social Policy* 44: 41–56.

Prévention CDN-NDG. 2019. *Cultivons la culture du consentement*. Montréal: Prévention CDN-NDG.

Puig de la Bellacasa, María. 2012. *Politiques féministes et construction des savoirs: "penser nous devons"!* Paris: L'Harmattan.

Rutherford, Alexandra. 2017a. B. F. Skinner and Technology's Nation: Technocracy, Social Engineering, and the Good Life in 20th-Century America. *History of Psychology* 20: 290–312. https://doi.org/10.1037/hop0000062.

Rutherford, Alexandra. 2017b. Surveying Rape: Feminist Social Science and the Ontological Politics of Sexual Assault. *History of the Human Sciences* 30: 100–123. https://doi.org/10.1177/0952695117722715.

Schneider, Elizabeth M. 2002. *Battered Women and Feminist Lawmaking*. New Haven: Yale University Press.

Staub, Michael, E. 2011. *Madness Is Civilization. When the Diagnosis was Social, 1948–1980*. Chicago: The University of Chicago Press.

Walker, Lenore E. 2009. *The Battered Woman Syndrome*, 3rd ed. New York: Springer.

Weber, M. (2017). *L'éthique protestante et l'esprit du capitalisme* (I. Kalinowski, Trans.). Flammarion.

Weidman, Nadine M. 2021. *Killer Instinct: The Popular Science of Human Nature in Twentieth-century America*. Cambridge, MA: Harvard University Press.

Weinstein, Deborah. 2013. *The Pathological Family: Postwar America and the Rise of Family Therapy*. Ithaca: Cornell University Press.

Weldon, S. Laurel. 2002. *Protest, Policy, and the Problem of Violence against Women*. Pittsburgh: University of Pittsburgh Press. https://doi.org/10.2307/j.ctt7zw85q.

Young, Allan. 1995. *The Harmony of Illusions: Inventing Post-Traumatic Stress Disorder*. Princeton, NJ Princeton University Press.

# Historical Perspectives on Prevention and Punishment of Child Sexual Abuse: Analysing Medico-Legal Responses

*Andy Kaladelfos and Lisa Featherstone*

## 1 Introduction

'Australia's Menace of the Prowling Pervert', read one headline of the popular and inexpensive Sydney newspaper *Truth* in 1925. The article pressured the government of New South Wales, the most populous state of Australia, to take action on sexual crimes against women and children. 'Segregation' was the only remedy for the problem, the newspaper opined, speaking not only of segregation within criminal justice institutions but also of social segregation, such as separate schools, for adolescents of those who exhibited what they saw as propensities for future crimes. Writing with little doubt on the cause of sexual crimes against children, the paper explained that:

A. Kaladelfos (✉)
University of New South Wales, Sydney, Australia
e-mail: a.kaladelfos@unsw.edu.au

L. Featherstone
University of Queensland, Brisbane, Australia
e-mail: l.featherstone@uq.edu.au



R. E. Keyse et al. (eds.), *Sexual Violence in Medicine and Psychiatry*, Genders and Sexualities in History,
https://doi.org/10.1007/978-3-032-10800-5_4

> [t]he clinical observer and psychologist know that the impelling motive for these atrocious and ruinous assaults on children of tender years ... is a twisted sort of perverted sexual desire ... These 'defectives' are easily detected by a clinical observer during school age (*Truth*, 15 February 1925).

To support their claims, the newspaper solicited the opinion of NSW parliamentarian Dr. Richard Arthur (1865–1932), a clinically trained medical doctor and president of the Eugenics Society of New South Wales. In parliament, Arthur regularly expressed the view that violent criminals belonged in mental institutions, not prisons. He told the paper that prisons were 'useless' as those who committed serious crimes against children were suffering from a form of insanity. The need for segregation of sexual offenders in a place of exclusion was 'one of the most pressing problems of the time'.

Arthur and *Truth's* perspectives were considered progressive and scientifically informed at the time. Their advocates positioned them in contrast to moral ideologies of sin or wrongdoing represented by imprisonment, corporal punishment, and capital punishment (Garton 2010).[1] The views were aired in the context of capital punishment being retained for rape and sexual offences on young girls in NSW and most states in Australia, unlike England, until well into the twentieth century (Kaladelfos 2012). After the turn of the century, and particularly in the interwar period, medical doctors, psychiatrists, and other scientifically trained theorists opposed capital, corporal, and prison punishment because they saw the mental treatment of those who committed serious crimes in line with scientific belief. Other proponents of policies of segregation and social isolation were less certain about the removal of older punishment styles, with women's advocacy groups and administrators of the criminal legal system maintaining they had a role in crime prevention and punishment. Both viewpoints–social segregation and prison punishment—formed an integral part of cultures of social exclusion and carcerality of the public health and criminal legal system (Bashford and Strange 2003).

In this chapter, we argue that medicine and psychiatry were important influences on the ideas about sexual offending and sexual offenders, showing the enmeshment of legal and medical opinion in forming the

[1] Corporal punishment was part of criminal legal punishments or a regime of punishments in schools or family homes, exempt from prosecution for criminal assault.

criminal legal and government responses to crime. Yet, just as importantly, we also highlight the complex interactions between experts and other groups in the community, to show how medical and legal opinion was absorbed, adapted, or challenged. We begin with a brief overview of the historical context, including legal and medical opinion, as well as the social and cultural milieu. Then, the chapter offers an analysis of public perceptions about sexual violence, and the impact of medicine, the law and socio-cultural factors on popular understandings across the decades. Throughout, we consider the impact of race, gender, and disability, and the ways that these interconnect with issues of sexual offending. Across the historical analysis, we seek to show that the mainstream perspectives on prevention and punishment of sexual offences which existed until at least the 1960s have ongoing resonances, and arguably continue to form the roots of contemporary criminal legal approaches to sexual offenders (Lussier et al. 2021; Smithers 2023).

## 2 Socio-legal Context

Child sexual abuse today is known to cause profound social and personal harm, with many victim-survivors experiencing lifelong traumatic after-effects of violence and social responses to abuse (Hailes et al. 2019). In contrast, in the early-to-mid twentieth century, there were far fewer concerns about psychological harm, and ideas of trauma were not commonly applied to victims of child sexual abuse. Instead, there were concerns over physical harm (including pregnancy), and social and economic harm (loss of virginity, or concerns over prospects for future marriage and family) (Featherstone 2018). For these reasons, some families felt that keeping abuse hidden may reduce the social impact or stigma on children, and in some instances extra-legal remedies such as the marriage to defendant in a rape case were supported by victim's families. Many others sought criminal legal remedies, with tens of thousands of child sexual abuse prosecutions before the 1960s in Australia (Finnane et al. 2023). With reckonings around the world of coverups about historical child sexual abuse in public and private institutions (Blakemore et al. 2017), past 'silence' has become a major framework for social understandings of historical conceptions of child sexual (Boxall et al. 2014). Historians have begun scholarly exchange on the history of child sexual abuse, which seeks to challenge this mythology and to explain historical perspectives on child sexual abuse more accurately (Basannavar 2018).

To understand the historical context, we briefly outline the background to four connecting socio-legal elements that were intertwined with medicine and psychiatric thought on sexual offending against children and its public dissemination: Australian criminal law; the position of expert evidence; public engagement on prevention and punishment of crime; and the influence of eugenic thought. This interconnected history of criminal law, social movements, punishment philosophies, and medical understandings of sexual violence has been an unappreciated aspect of the history of child sexual offences (Kaladelfos and Piper 2022). After we examine this context, we highlight key turning points, statutory or procedural development, and social ideas about child sexual offences in the decades until the 1960s.

From the late nineteenth century, the sexual assault of children was understood as a social and moral problem with remedies offered within the law, state institutions, communities, and households. Remedies focused on retributive punishment and crime prevention for child sexual abuse was an indirect concept, imagined to be achieved by increasing the moral and social standing of future citizens through their discipline as children, including religious observance, work, family units and cultural norms of respectability, virtue, and honour. There was very little proactive policing for sexual offences on children—except for occasional crackdowns on young women's sexual behaviour—with most offences coming to the notice of police after reports from victim's families or community members. From the 1920s onwards, medicine, psychiatry and psychology increasingly intervened in understanding criminality, albeit with varying degrees of acceptance by judges presiding over criminal sentencing. While these perspectives varied in their moral, behavioural, and biological focus, practitioners continued to refer to all three aspects blurring the lines between so-called traditional and modern punishment ideologies. Punishment became more focused on rehabilitation, or what is termed in criminology 'tertiary' prevention (after a crime).

At the same time, government interest in crime prevention increased. These ideas of prevention were understood in a number of ways. At a population level, rudimentary sex education was increased, to focus the young mind on 'healthy' normative heterosexuality (Featherstone 2011). There was also a new focus on medicalisation, including the physiological and psychological screening of young people. Alongside the medical turn, there was an increased police presence, especially by the 1950s, to proactively monitor the sexual behaviour of all citizens. Increased policing was tied to both prevention and punishment, for example in child welfare regimes (Featherstone and Kaladelfos 2016). Like contemporary understandings of prevention and punishment there was a close entanglement, with the state promoting and utilising both prevention and policing in an attempt to control offending and social norms.

### 2.1 *Child Sexual Abuse and Criminal Law*

In Australian jurisdictions, most states maintained a death sentence for rape of any woman, 'carnal knowledge' (an equivalent of rape) of a young girl—the young age being variously defined as under the age of 10, 12, or 13 in different jurisdictions—long after England had removed them from criminal law in 1841 (Kaladelfos 2012). There were just over 500 men sentenced to death for sexual offences after that period, and c.125 men in the twentieth century (Finnane et al. 2023). As the capital punishment abolitionist movement gained traction in the late nineteenth century, executions for sexual offences were increasingly a target of public agitation, with many critiquing why colonies maintained harsher criminal laws than that of England. The argument colonial lawmakers put forward to justify it was that white women and girls needed 'protection'. This rhetoric had different elements regionally: in NSW, concerns were about white ex-convict men in the bush and Aboriginal men, whereas in Queensland, colonised 70 years after NSW, white colonists targeted criminal legal responses to Aboriginal men and South Sea Islander men in the most racially targeted use of executions in Australian history. Despite that history, Queensland was the first state to abolish the death penalty for rape and carnal knowledge offences in 1899.

The last known use of these provisions in Australia was the 1932 execution of David Robert Bennett in the state of Victoria. Bennett was a white man with a long criminal record, including a previous child sexual abuse conviction and a life sentence in Western Australia in 1911 (*Western Star* 1932; *Prosecution Project* [*PP*], Trial ID #3280). He was executed for the serious sexual assault of a 4-year-old girl. Unlike his contemporaries in the nineteenth century, there was little public abolitionist support for Bennett. Activism was mostly reserved for organised political groups: the Victorian Trades Hall Council in Melbourne and the Victorian branch of the 'Howard League for Penal Reform', headed by Scottish minister Charles Strong. The Howard League urged the Victorian government to impose a life imprisonment sentence instead following 'the spirit and principle of modern psychology and penology', explaining that 'Crime, we feel, cannot by such vengeful methods be up-rooted, nor sexual insanity be diminished' (Strong 1932).

By the early twentieth century, every Australian state had developed additional age-based offences for 'carnal knowledge' and 'indecent assault'. Most jurisdictions had provisions for age-based offences on girls and boys, whereas NSW was alone in not creating separate age-based offences for offences on boys. These offences could be used for the policing of prohibited consensual sex amongst young people, but far more often used to prosecute what we would understand to be aggravated rape or sexual abuse violations. Some Australian jurisdictions maintained unique provisions criminalising teacher's sexual assault of their pupils, and South Australia was amongst the first in the world to introduce incest provisions (Kaladelfos and Featherstone 2016; Kaladelfos 2019).

### 2.2 *Role of Medical Expertise*

Australian jurisdictions did not uniformly adopt notable international innovations in sexual psychiatry in legal regulation or courtroom practice. In Canada and the United States, by the mid-twentieth century, medical science and psychiatric testimony were central to statutory and regulatory approaches to the prevention and punishment of sexual offences. From the 1930s, North American jurisdictions introduced legislation to deal with sexual offences that linked the legal system to health care, positioning the sexual 'pervert' as a mental disorder that could be treated by psychiatry. Some states could (and still can) hold a person convicted of serious sexual crimes for an indefinite period, purportedly to prevent reoffending and for the psychiatric treatment of the offender (Chenier 2003; Freedman 1989; Chauncey 1993; Terry 2007). Similar models existed in two Australian jurisdictions (Tasmania and Queensland) by the early 1950s but appear to have been used very little (PP, TASSC; PP, QLDSC). Judges in all states could request medical evidence at sentencing, but this was not routine, and most judges did not readily accept the medical evidence produced by psychiatrists seeing it as unreliable science. By the mid-twentieth century, psychiatric evidence was increasingly challenging the use of retributive punishments, although the courts were slow to change. Judges often used discretionary sentencing in terms of the length of imprisonment and an increase in suspended sentences, but were reluctant to completely dissolve conventional retributive options (Featherstone and Kaladelfos 2016).

### 2.3 *Eugenics, Race and Disability*

If, in criminal sentencing, psychiatry had less impact than might be expected, medicalised views were apparent in the wider community, in particular through the pseudo-science of eugenics. Eugenic beliefs had a significant impact on almost every aspect of Australian social life and political life in this time period. Eugenic influence is most readily apparent in the genocidal policies that created the Stolen Generations—the decades-long policies to remove Aboriginal children from their families and their placement in reservations that were designed to 'breed out the colour' (McGregor 2002). The vision of Australia as a white nation, and active social engineering of population was evident in the 'White Australia' immigration policy, which created several prohibited migration categories. The unwritten prohibition based on race is the most well-known, where a dictation test was used to prohibit entry of non-Anglo immigrants. The Act's other prohibitions were equally important, including restrictions on potential immigrant's mental and physical health and criminal history. These issues were grounds for denial of entry and deportation of those who were not citizens, both heavily connected to the history of disability and the criminal legal system's reach and common elsewhere in the Anglophone world (Lira 2021; Baynton 2016).

Views like Arthur's and *Truth's* at the outset of this chapter were entwined with eugenic thinking. While commentators on child sexual abuse did not necessarily make the specific link, ideas about criminality were imbued with eugenic thinking. It was believed that both the prevention and punishment of child sexual abuse could ultimately be achieved through deliberative social engineering—ideas that remained even after the decline of eugenics following the Second World War. Children should be screened, some argued, for medical and mental 'defects' and 'segregated' or 'treated', sometimes through interventions such as sterilisation, often proposed for sexual crimes (Evans 2017; Evans and Parry 2001). These approaches were thought to limit an individuals' future offending and thereby stop the creation of future generations with 'defective' genes and psyches. Eugenic beliefs directly influenced policies on juvenile 'delinquency', a category that would now be seen as at the cross-roads of juvenile justice and mental health interventions, and in particular, eugenics had profound impacts on reproduction and population policy. These were most directly felt in Tasmania which was unique in the fact that it attempted to impose a government-organised screening process to identify 'deficiency' within schools.[2]

## 2.4 *Popular Punitivism*

While there was widespread public support for eugenic thinking (at least until World War II), and a belief in the need for high-level surveillance over reproduction, including the reproduction of criminality, when it came to individual offenders, public interest remained focused on offender-based prevention and punishment of child sexual abuse. An offender was perceived to be as identifiable through biological, social or moral attributes. At the same time, there was little emphasis on victim-oriented advocacy, victim-survivor experiences of the justice system, or education-focused primary prevention, at least until they gained some traction amongst women's movements (Blewer 2021). But the main focus of advocacy was concerns over the punishment of sexual offenders. Criminologists would recognise these concepts as relating to the 'popular punitivism' towards sexual offences often traced back to 'signal' crimes in the 1990s and 2000s (McAlinden 2014). The origins of these views are much longer—historians have shown there were many earlier examples of 'sex murders' in the 1920s-1940s, that were also viewed as signal crimes at the time (Strange 2018, 2020). Public perceptions of sexual offending, particularly conservative women's perceptions, have long influenced political and policy approaches. To do this, women's groups drew on medical and pseudo-medical language to propose punishments that were not always cohesive to a particular theoretical position about crime's origins. For example, many proponents were staunchly in favour of capital punishment as well as medical intervention. As the rest of this chapter will show, public perceptions about child sexual abuse were influenced by a raft of factors, some legal, some medical, and others social and cultural. The next sections trace the broad differences across the decades, to show the changes and continuities in understandings of and attitudes towards child sexual abuse and the treatments and responses it required.

[2] 'Deficiency' was a broad category, sometimes about a diagnosable medical condition such as epilepsy or a more malleable category such as 'moral' disorder.

## 3 1920s: Public Mobilisation

In the early 1920s, a series of serious sexual assaults and killings of young children saw the start of organised medical and social responses to sex offending that went far beyond medical interventions proposed in other forms of non-sexual offending. Amongst these were several sex-related killings: the murder of a 13-year-old girl in a regional area of Tasmania in 1921, the murder of a 12-year-old girl in Melbourne in 1922, the manslaughter case of a 5-year-old boy in Sydney in 1923, and the murder of an 11-year-old Melbourne girl in 1924 (*Advocate* 1921; *Age* 1922; *Daily Telegraph* 1923; *Herald* 1924). Each case attracted significant public interest and medical testimony, and some remain unsolved. Tasmanian women were amongst the most organised: following the 1921 murder, they arranged multiple meetings with the Attorney General representing the 'Women's Association for Criminal Law Reform' (*Examiner* 20 June 1921). Specifically positioning themselves as educated and concerned women of the state, they sought 'indefinite sentences' for men convicted of sexual crimes, regarding them as 'abnormal and dangerous to society'. Soon after, the Tasmanian government passed legislation relating to indeterminate sentences, although there was no specific reference to sexual offences until some decades later (Tasmania 1921).

Before the First World War, medical thought shifted towards examining the aetiology of criminal offending. While views were mixed on whether criminality itself was considered a sign of mental disease or even 'insanity', the leading Australian medical journal published editorials in the 1910s and 1920s around this issue, endorsing the use of medical tribunals instead of juries or judges to decide upon criminal outcomes (Lind 1916). The concerns were generally split between what they considered prevention or rehabilitation initiatives, with an earlier focus on the first and later on the second. An editorial piece in the 1920 edition of the premier medical journal outlined what authors considered a medically appropriate remedy for crime: that screening for mental defectiveness should occur for each person convicted (Editors, *Medical Journal of Australia* [henceforth MJA] 1920). For those deemed 'normal', a long imprisonment sentence should be imposed, while recidivists who were deemed 'normal' should receive a life sentence. It was one of the most 'serious blots' on the social system, the author lamented, that the law does not differentiate between 'normal' criminals and mentally deficient. In the second category, the editorial proposed a system of home and school screening and the use of medical psychiatrists at trial to decide whether a person was defective or not. What should happen to those found to be mentally defective was less clear: it was simply described as a system of 'permanent control'. Later editorials in the journal praised the Tasmanian government system of mental deficiency screening in schools and the grading and segregation of those deemed of a lower mental condition, describing a system of early recognition as 'Utopian conditions'. The editors believed that utilising both psychiatry and psychology would be the best approach and that these medical areas should be embedded in prisons (Editors, *MJA* 1927). In essence, the medical approach to child sexual abuse was not independent from the criminal legal punishment and its carceral intent, though as we have noted, the two were not as co-dependent as in North America, where practice routinely intertwined the criminal and the medical.

The 1920s was the decade that saw the mobilisation of white, middle-class conservative women's groups, often with eugenic philosophies around the issues of sexual offences against children, which continued for decades (Petrow 1995). As the decades passed, women's organisations continued to draw on medical, psychiatric, *and* moral ideologies of prevention and punishment to persuade governments to introduce forms of social control in crime prevention and punishment. Sometimes, these aspects were towards the same ends: for example, segregation aimed to incapacitate and reduce the 'contamination' of other people in closed institutions. Their perspectives were informed by medical thinking, but they also fervently argued for punishments on the body, especially corporal punishment, a constant element of their advocacy. The 1920s saw a clear jostling for authority to speak on criminal offending matters between legal actors and medical professionals. Medical doctors were gradually asserting their superiority, as they saw it, in determining who was and who wasn't a danger to society.

## 4 1930s: Institutional Investigations

In 1934, William George Lincoln (pseudonym) had just turned 18 when he pleaded guilty to committing two counts of indecent assault against young boys while he was an inmate of a youth detention facility. Presiding over his sentencing was Judge Curlewis of the Quarter Sessions (a mid-level court), who reported that earlier evidence had been given that while Lincoln was under the age of 18, he had been flogged for the offence in the children's home. Officials denied corporal punishment, insisting he was punished by deprivation of food (bread and water only) on a single occasion. After he turned 18, he was turned over to police (*Sun* 1934; *Sydney Morning Herald* 1934).

The detention centre, in Gosford, a regional area outside Sydney, had been originally modelled on progressive beliefs of reformation: a semi-rural property, with nature and trades that would facilitate useful citizenry amongst its detainees (Find and Connect n.d.). Over the decades of its running, the enforcement of discipline became increasingly brutal, including the use of older inmates acting as 'styled junior officers' to punish younger children—a practice criticised by a major government inquiry into juvenile detention facilities that year. It was within this culture—senior boys monitoring younger ones that—that Lincoln had been abusing children (New South Wales 1934).

We do not learn of these circumstances of Lincoln's abuse either from his sentencing or the government inquiry. Instead, the records come from within the New South Wales Department of Prisons, which, in the early 1930s, began recording the case histories of men who committed sexual offences, most of them on children (State Records NSW, c. 1935). These short narrations, existing in a hand-written and undated volume, provide a window into medico-legal concern over sexual offences in the period between the two world wars. Lincoln's narration was one of the longest in the series, with around 200 case histories taken in total. Lincoln's history explained that his offences occurred while he was a 'monitor on night duty' when he took children who had wet the bed to the lavatory. Lincoln's case history contained two previous sexual offences on young girls, aged 6 and 8 and committed when he was a minor, the current conviction and a report from Dr. E.S. Holloway, a visiting surgeon at Long Bay Gaol. Holloway noted that Lincoln knew the difference between right and wrong but had a mental age of about 12–13 and little 'self-control'.

Neither Holloway, an experienced prison doctor, nor Judge Curlewis, who had presided over hundreds of criminal trials by this time, knew how to sentence Lincoln. Curlewis, like other judges who would come after him, remained dissatisfied with the options, or lack thereof, telling Lincoln that he was imprisoning him because there was no other treatment available. Dr. Holloway provided a longer explanation: 'punitive treatment' has done little or nothing in his case, outlining the available medical options (State Records NSW, c. 1935). First considering a surgical treatment ('castration'), but offered the view that there was little current medical evidence to support it. He believed that Lincoln was 'a suitable case for permanent detention in an institution for the mentally defective'. At sentencing, Curlewis noted that Lincoln was a 'menace to little boys and girls' but that prison was the only option available, sentencing Lincoln to two years (*Sun* 1934). The last known record of Lincoln's interactions with the justice system was when he was released on licence (a type of parole) in 1936.

By this point, technologies of detection by police had developed to contain hundreds of narrative 'modus operandi' reports. Upon release on licence, these were printed in police gazettes that circulated around the state photos, case histories, and brief descriptions such as height and distinguishing features. Many contain quasi-medical conclusions and presumptions, where medical jargon was utilised by people who were not medical professionals, and who did not necessarily apply the specific scientific meanings of words or diagnoses. Further, even medical professionals could draw loosely on categorisation which had cultural, not merely medical, meanings. In the modus operandi report, Lincoln was described as a 'sexual maniac', of 'dull intellect', 'morally depraved', and a 'definite menace to children' (NSW Police 1936). The denotation 'sexual maniac' was one of many loose psy-terminologies used before the 1970s to describe men who abused children. This terminology was generally used to describe serious sexual offences, like other terminologies such as 'sexual degenerate', 'sexual offenders', and often with the broadest meaning 'sexual pervert', as well as various similarly broad terms for the mentally ill, especially 'mental defective'. In the 1936 NSW Police Gazette, Lincoln was the only person described as a sexual maniac, whereas another six people were described as a sexual pervert (often those with a mixed offending history: for example, 'thief, pretender and sexual pervert'), and a further nine people described as a 'sexual offender'. These terms drifted between scientific and social meanings and were far from homogenous. Of those noted to have a sexual offending history, the circumstances varied from rape offences, familial child sexual abuse, indecent exposure, attempted abduction of a woman, and a smaller number of cases in line with the criminalisation of homosexuality.

The examples throughout the 1930s show the reach of medical and psychological terminologies and concepts across different technologies and tracking systems of policing and punishment. These technologies—earlier examples of typologies that would later be developed through police such as in the FBI—showed several important things. First is the scientific and professional interest scale and investment of resources in cataloguing sex offenders. Second, the widespread knowledge that sex offenders had both specific and versatile profiles, and that some offenders targeted children. We might call this decade one of 'exploration': state officials were focused on surveillance, categorisation, and monitoring of a well-known social and policy problem, highlighting the intersections between medicine and criminal justice when considering offences against children.

While the criminal legal institutions, especially prisons, were producing their own exploration of the issue of sexual offenders, women's associations were increasing their campaigns for punitive measures. Archival materials show persistent women's lobbying on the punishments handed down for crimes against children. From the mid-1930s onwards, the New South Wales Attorney General's Department maintained dedicated files on reporting and correspondence on sexual offenders, many of them from conservative women's organisations (State Records NSW 1919–1945). Ms. Lilian Price, the General Secretary of the Country Women's Association of NSW, regularly corresponded with the Attorney General's department about resolutions the association had made about sexual offenders. In 1934, writing that one local Sydney branch carried the resolution that a Bill should be provided 'for the sterilisation of person convicted of debasing sex crimes upon children of tender years' and later argued for 'segregation' (in 1938 and 1943). In 1937 she wrote to the justice department that the organisation had passed a resolution in favour of the use of corporal punishment for sexual offenders, which they felt would 'act as a deterrent', and in 1941, advising that one local association had passed a resolution in favour of the use of capital punishment for 'sexual outrages against children'. Other groups, such as Parents and Citizens' Association groups from local schools, regularly wrote to the government with similar proposals. In 1946, the Housewives Association of NSW Chairman of Directors, Mrs. Eleanor Glencross, wrote to the minister of justice outlining a resolution from her association that corporal punishment be introduced, a psychiatrist used to 'deal with' cases of sexual offences on women and children, and for repeat offenders 'segregated for life'.

These views were connected to those regularly espoused by the Racial Hygiene Association. In 1938, Mrs. L. E. Goddisson, the general secretary of the Association, called for segregation to 'reduce the number of outrages on children', contrasting them to 'punitive' measures, which they said have not worked. The association believed that courts should have the benefits of judges, psychiatrists, and social workers. They connected child sexual offences to 'deficient children', noting that farm colonies should be introduced from a young age. Although these views were not uniform, with other lesser-known women's groups writing to the government to assert that corporal punishment was a 'convict day' remnant, and medical and psychological thought would deem temporary or permanent segregation of sexual offenders to be the most modern course of action. Across the 1930s, then, there were numerous layers of thinking about child sex abuse, all of which brought new, 'scientific' modes of thinking to the problem of criminal offending.

## 5 1940s: Regulatory Frameworks

From the late 1930s to the mid-1940s, attention turned to legislative or other forms of government intervention in controlling, segregating, and monitoring men with sexual offending histories. NSW eventually passed regulations around 1939, which provided far-reaching controls for medical examination of prisons and referrals to courts for institutionalisation (New South Wales 1939). Although the debates and public discussion around the introduction of this legislation were strongly focused on sexual offences and crimes against children, the Act as made was broad and not focused on any specific offence. It also specified 'a visiting surgeon' or 'medical practitioner' rather than a psychiatrist as those making decisions about prisoners, unlike other state's regulations.

In 1940, South Australia was the first Australian state to develop specific provisions for punishing sexual offenders. The *Criminal Law Consolidation Act 1940 (SA)* developed a provision that for any person guilty of a sexual offence, a judge could order at their discretion two or more medical practitioners to examine whether the offender was 'incapable of exercising proper control over his sexual instincts'. If the medical practitioners reported an incapability, the court could issue an indeterminate sentence at the Governor's discretion. The Act contained similar provisions if the medical reports deemed the offender capable but with 'subnormal' medical conditions. Practically, both options could result in indefinite detention. The same Act also prescribed indeterminate sentences in the case of sexual offenders with venereal diseases. The correlation of discussions around sexual offenders with venereal disease prevention and control was a talking point regularly used by the Racial

Hygiene Society: the eugenicist society had previously proposed that a specialist court be created on the issue of criminal responsibility, headed by a mental health expert, a venereal disease specialist and a doctor (*Telegraph*, 6 October 1933).

During WWII, with tens of thousands of American troops populating the shores of Queensland, the Attorney-General set about appointing a Committee to engage in questions of sexual offences and punishment systems. The committee had nine terms of reference: to examine the prevalence of specific offences on women and children and whether they had increased; to consider whether the offences were the results of 'mental perversion', 'abnormality', or 'mental sickness'; to find on whether current punishments were adequate or if measures such as 'segregation' or 'physical, mental, surgical' treatment were required; and to consider any preventative measures with an offender focus. Sitting for 15 days, the committee heard evidence from women's organisations for child safety; superintendents of juvenile delinquency homes; police officers; and medical professionals. In 1944, the QLD parliament tabled a significant inquiry into the treatment of sexual offences, confining its remit to sexual offences on women and children. The following year, a successful Act in Queensland saw the creation of provisions in the *Criminal Law Amendment Act* 1945: An Act for the 'Treatment and Punishment of Offenders convicted of Sexual Offences'. This Act created provisions for indeterminate sentences outside long-existing lunacy provisions (usually involving a case where one was determined not to be fit to plead to an offence or after being determined not criminally responsible for a crime). The 1945 Act was unusual in that it didn't relate sexual offending to criminal responsibility but effectively to dangerousness to the public. The Act set out that in any case involving a sexual offence on a person under 17, a judge or magistrate could ask two medical doctors, one being a psychiatrist, to decide whether the prisoner was 'capable' of 'controlling sex instincts'. If their recommendation was negative, the judge could recommend indefinite detention: that is, at the 'Governor's Pleasure'.

While criminology regularly explains theories of punishment in broad brush strokes (a move from punishment on the body to the mind using Foucauldian paradigms), the administration of the mid-twentieth-century criminal legal system held both aspects hand-in-hand. The medical model did not preclude the use, in symbolism and practice, of punishments on the body. The very same South Australian amendment in 1940 that introduced the possibility of medical advice and models applied to sexual offenders, also specified the punishment of whipping for carnal knowledge offences. The persistent use of corporal punishment as a remedy of sexual offenders was a belief held at some of the highest levels of justice administration.

For instance, Joseph Akeroyd, the Victorian Inspector-General of Prisons for almost two decades declared that psychiatric concepts of dealing with sexual offenders were 'pure unadulterated hooey', notwithstanding that he had overseen the development of a system of segregation in Victorian prisons using psychological and psychiatric concepts (*Herald* 1947). Akeroyd went on to explain that he preferred whipping sexual offenders as it 'led a man to think'. Whipping, generally seen to have a deterrent function, in 1947 was extolled as preparing men for the 'positive measures of reform' (*Daily Mercury* 1947; Wilson 2014). Whipping, then, was imagined as both a preventative and a punishment. Giving evidence to a Victorian law reform committee on the question of retaining physical punishments (capital and corporal), Akeroyd answered a question about sexual crimes against young girls. He explained:

There are sex crimes and there are sex crimes. There are some in which the offender is not definitely a pathological case. A pathological case should never be whipped, but there are some offenders who are not pathological. They are men like you and me but who have never been trained to decent conduct. They could well be pulled up by a whipping. (Victoria 1948).

Akeroyd's perspective dominated many of the ideologies held by those administering the criminal legal system: that there was a distinction between medically diagnosable and immoral behaviours. Akeroyd went further than most, suggesting that any man could be a sexual offender depending on education and training. This went to the heart of some prevention beliefs: that sexual violence resulted from sexual or immoral impulses and could, therefore, be treated with restorative examples or punishments.

Even John Catarinich, the Director of Mental Health Institutions in Victoria, was similarly circumspect about the role and utility of psychiatric measures for sexual offenders. Writing in the 1944 Annual Report, he noted that public sentiment often accepted that 'modern methods' would 'change the personality of sex perverts and by so doing turn them into normal members of society'. He went on to say while this may be true in some instances and medical assessment should occur for all sexual offenders, but he was worried about overblowing psychiatric assertions of a 'cure' for sexual offending. He was concerned about the growing tendency of Victorian courts to refer cases to the mental health department when the prisoner may not be suitable for any treatment or may still bear responsibility for the crime (Victoria 1944). Here, we see the tensions between the various models of understanding sexual criminality, and the ways that those in authority attempted to navigate them, a problem that continued in coming decades.

## 6 1950s: Mainstreaming Medical Approaches

The smallest state of Tasmania in 1951 introduced a specific legislative framework in dealing with the treatment of sexual offenders, following the Queensland Act formulated as the 'protection of women and children'. *The Sexual Offences Act* 1951 (Tas) empowered the Director of Mental Hygiene to detain any person who has confessed or been found guilty of a sexual offence and to be examined 'using force' if necessary by three medical examiners: one doctor, one psychiatrist and one psychologist, to order treatment or segregation of the prisoner. But despite the introduction of new provisions, the Tasmanian segregation system appears to have been only used a limited number of times after its inception. Based upon the Tasmanian register of criminal indictments, only four instances to the end of the 1950s were found (two relating to homosexual offences and two to offences on children [*PP*, TASSC]). These findings accord with prior studies: research on the designation of 'habitual criminals' which showed that it was far more likely to be used for robbery offences; and research on the 1950s found very sparing use of indefinite detention provisions (such as mental defectives acts) (Durnian 2021; Featherstone and Kaladelfos 2016). While it is possible that interventions occurred before or post-sentencing, from the criminal law perspective, it was more symbolic rather than comprehensive.

In criminal legal processes, most commonly, psychiatrists were called to give evidence at sentencing hearings, with the court relying on a small number of specialists who worked with prison populations and were generally experienced with courtroom testimony. These psychiatrists generally met briefly once or twice with the prisoner while he was in gaol before sentencing, using an interview to attempt to establish a commentary on his background, family life and mental capacity. Comprehensive and rigorous psychiatric testing was rarely utilised and was generally deployed by doctors working in private practice rather than those in the public sector.[3]

As psychiatric evidence almost always came into play at sentencing, it was generally presented before a judge, rather than the jury. By the 1950s, the reception of psychiatric evidence depended on the judge's attitude towards medical testimony and treatment, and this could vary widely between individual judges. In New South Wales the Quarter Sessions Judge Frederick Berne often enthusiastically engaged with psychiatric evidence. In his courtroom, Judge Berne gave a great deal of earnest consideration to psychiatric testimony, and he engaged with medical theories of sexology, pathology and deviance. Berne actively sought out expert testimony of psychiatrists, noting in one trial in 1953 that 'with sexual offenders I like to ascertain from an expert—I want advice really before I deal with them' (State Records NSW 1953a, b). Berne noted that sexual offenders varied in their offences; treatment; recidivism; and the possibility of a cure. As such, he preferred to consult medical staff, and to carefully consider the psychiatric and sexological evidence presented. He went so far as to note in one case: 'I am not a psychiatrist; how can I refuse to accept the doctor's evidence (State Records NSW 1954)?'.

But even Berne did not always accept psychiatric evidence. In 1953, when a man indecently assaulted a seven-year-old girl, Berne was scathing at even considering medical treatment: 'no medical treatment as yet known to science can do anything to curb your evil tendencies, vicious tendencies, and certainly not cure you' (State Records NSW 1953b). Similarly in 1958, Max Thymes pleaded guilty to four counts of indecent assault on a male, where the victim was a ten-year-old boy. Thymes had a long list of priors for sexual assault and had seen significant gaol time during the 1940s and 1950s. The defence attorney requested the Judge appoint a court ordered psychiatrist to examine Thymes, but the Judge refused, stating that his recidivism showed that he continued to be a 'menace' to young boys, whatever the medical evidence might indicate (State Records NSW 1958).

While some psychiatrists believed men could be coaxed from homosexuality into normative heterosexuality, it was clear that medicine or psychiatric care was highly contested as a 'cure' for other sexual offences

[3] More comprehensive testing by doctors in the public sector may have occurred after incarceration, while in the prison population. See Featherstone and Kaladelfos, *Sex Crimes in the Fifties*, 178–82.

in mid-century Australia (Featherstone 2017). Some were even actively opposed to psychiatric intervention. For example, a member of the Victorian Indeterminate Sentences Board argued that medical intervention was not productive for those who committed sex offences: 'When they go before psychiatrists it boosts their ego ... Sex offenders can put it over psychiatrists 99 per cent of the time'. This expert indicated his support for the reintroduction of birching in Victoria, which had recently been removed (*Advocate* 1953). Thus even as doctors were consolidated as part of the criminal justice sector, their interventions were frequently not valued and their expertise undermined.

## 7 1960s: Institutional Frameworks

The relationships between medicine, policing and the courts continued to be obscure, in practice as well as policy. For example, annual reports from mental illness facilities were often opaque in indicating whether admissions had resulted from criminal offending and, even less so, what offences to which they were related. The place of sexual offending in admissions was often not clear. Medical professionals, lawmakers, and public engagement regularly pointed to alternative modes of carcerality, such as the use of indefinite sentences via institutionalisation, which shows the direct relationship between psychiatry and the justice sector. Yet there was little transparency on how prevalent this usage had become in the mid-twentieth century. A research article published by Herbert Bower, a psychiatrist at Kew Mental Hospital in Melbourne, in 1960 sheds light on the prevalence of institutional detention. Bower's research cross-referenced criminal offence categories to mental health conditions, showing that of the 122 men and women detained in Victorian mental asylums for criminal offences, 20 were detained for sex-related offences. This was not the largest category. The two larger were homicide (25) and vagrancy (22), although it is possible that both those categories may have contained offences adjacent to sexual violence. Of the 20 cases identified, 13 were held for 'mental deficiency', the largest single category. The other categories were 5 for 'schizophrenic' disorder, one for mental deficiency and 'psychosis' and a further one for the ambiguous diagnosis of 'character disorder'. Considering Victorian higher courts in this period heard over 200 prosecutions for sexual offences per year and homicide cases around 35, the number of those detained in mental health institutions for sexual offences alone are relatively small in comparison (Bower 1960; *PP*, VICSC 1956).

Forensic psychiatrists like Bower increasingly engaged with local and international medical texts (Editors, *MJA* 1948, 1950; McGeorge 1950, 1954). The NSW chief government psychiatrist John McGeorge, for instance, produced two key treatises on child sexual assault and broader sexual pathologies in the 1960s, which meticulously listed various forms of sexual deviation (1964, 1966). In 1964, in the British publication of the Academy for Forensic Science *Medicine, Science and the Law*, he published an overview of British and American scientific literature on child sexual abuse, including paedophilia, and the results of decades of clinical observation during his role as chief psychiatrist at Long Bay Gaol, in Sydney. In contrast to earlier conceptions of sexual crimes against children, the taxonomy of sexual offenders was by now more developed. McGeorge explained various pathologies that could influence offending, which varied from the 'psychopath', 'psychotic', 'epileptic', 'alcoholic' to the 'homo-sexual' and 'paedophile'. In this paper, he continued his earlier conflation of homosexuality and paedophilia, pronouncing that there was a significant correlation between the two dispositions. He went on to explain that the pathology of the paedophile should be 'distinguished from the depraved type for whom the defencelessness of the child has an appeal'. The article went on to enumerate particular behaviours observed in clinical cases of child sexual abuse that he had advised on, devoting a long section to counting what he described as the 'co-operation' of children in their abuse (McGeorge 1964). These sections reveal the deep-seated contradictions within medical science. Though experts were increasingly recognising pathology, and the troubling impact of child sexual abuse, many still believed in crime prevention as a moral pursuit, where good citizens, including children, should be protected. Even a psychiatrist such as McGeorge—who had treated hundreds of men with sexual pathologies—could still readily defer to a moral agenda when discussing the socio-medical apparatus of sexual offending.

## 8 Conclusion

Examining the evolution of medical knowledge and transmission across four decades, we contend that social knowledge about child sexual abuse has been a serious concern of government, which developed concurrently and, in some ways, preceded clinical medical understanding of specific pathologies. In this chapter, we have delineated the interactions between medical and legal authorities over four decades, and how these intersected with popular understandings. We have contextualised historical understanding of child sexual abuse amidst criminal legal responses, the prevalence of eugenic discourses and programmes, and the lack of trust of psychiatric cures. The development of a large institutional apparatus for indefinite sentences and the implementation of specific legislative provisions in several jurisdictions starkly contrasted the lack of use of these provisions. We show that both moralistic views on crime prevention and retributive punishments retained significant sway amongst public advocates and experts who were not yet (or not ever perhaps) persuaded by the value of an exclusive medicalised model. Close examination of these contexts challenges histories that date the development of ideas around child sexual offending to the existence of medicalised models (Angelides 2005), showing that since at least the 1920s there was significant exchange between women's organisations, lawmakers, and specialists in responding to the problem of child sexual abuse.

**Funding** This research was supported by Australian Research Council Discovery Projects DP190100322 and DP230101503. The authors declare no competing interests.

## References

### Primary Material

Australia's Menace of the Prowling Pervert. *Truth* (Sydney), 15 February 1925.

Birch for sexual offences' plea. *Advocate*, 18 April 1953. http://nla.gov.au/nla.news-article69468006. Accessed on 18 September 2024.

Bower, H. M. 1960. The Hospitalization of the 'Criminal Insane' in Victoria. *Medical Journal of Australia (MJA)* 2: 41–47. https://doi.org/10.5694/j.1326-5377.1960.tb86965.x.

Criminal Law Reform. *Examiner*, 20 June 1921. http://nla.gov.au/nla.news-article51129979. Accessed on 18 September 2024.

Colin Ross Guilty. *Age*, 27 February 1922. http://nla.gov.au/nla.news-article205748739. Accessed on 18 September 2024.

Child's Death. *Daily Telegraph*, 12 September 1923. http://nla.gov.au/nla.news-article246057805. Accessed on 18 September 2024.

Editors. 1920. Crimes and Criminals. *Medical Journal of Australia,* 5 June.

Editors. 1927. Criminology and Mental Deficiency. *Medical Journal of Australia,* 16 April.

Editors. 1948. Homosexuality. *Medical Journal of Australia,* 7 February.

Editors. 1950. Sexual Psychopathy. *Medical Journal of Australia,* 9 September.

Gaol Term. *Sun,* 12 July 1934. http://nla.gov.au/nla.news-article229563812. Accessed on 18 September 2024.

Lad Flogged. *Sun,* 3 July 1934. http://nla.gov.au/nla.news-article229568292. Accessed on 18 September 2024.

Lind, W.A.T. 1916. Criminology as Branch of Medicine. *Medical Journal of Australia,* 8 July.

McGeorge, J. 1950. Sexual Maladjustment in Neuropathic Personality. *Medical Journal of Australia,* 25 March.

McGeorge, J. 1954 Medico-Legal Aspects of Psychiatry. *Medical Journal of Australia,* 30 October.

McGeorge, J. 1964. Sexual Assaults on Children. *Medicine Science and the Law* 4: 245–253.

McGeorge, J. 1966. *Reflections of a Psychiatrist.* Sydney: Hodder & Stoughton.

Mrs. Tuckerman's Hope. *Herald,* 17 October 1924. http://nla.gov.au/nla.news-article244850342. Accessed on 18 September 2024.

Much Psychiatric Evidence Pure Hooey, Says Gaols Head. *Herald,* 18 October 1947. http://nla.gov.au/nla.news-article243566900. Accessed on 18 September 2024.

New South Wales. 1939. *Mental Defectives (Convicted Persons) Act.*

New South Wales, Parliament. 1934. *Child Welfare Report,* Legislative Assembly.

New South Wales Police. 1936. *Criminal Register Supplement (Police Gazette),* 17 June, entry 147, np.

*Prosecution Project.* 1932. Trial ID #3280, Victorian Supreme Court [VICSC], David Robert Bennett.

*Prosecution Project.* 1950–59. Tasmanian Supreme Court [TASSC] Registers of Indictment.

*Prosecution Project.* 1950–59. Queensland Supreme Court [QLDSC] Registers of Indictment.

Quarter Sessions. *Sydney Morning Herald,* 13 July 1934. http://nla.gov.au/nla.news-article17087560. Accessed on 18 September 2024.

Racial Hygiene. *Telegraph,* 6 October 1933. http://nla.gov.au/nla.news-article180592566. Accessed on 18 September 2024.

State Records NSW. c.1935. Corrective Services, *Record of Sexual Offenders,* NRS-1879, 5/1101, 89–90.

State Records NSW. 1919–45. Attorney General Special Bundles 'Sexual Offenders', 12/1351.1, various correspondence.

State Records NSW. 1953a. Court Reporting Branch; NRS 2713, Criminal Transcripts [hereafter Criminal Transcripts], Quarter Sessions, *R v Elms*.

State Records NSW. 1953b. Criminal Transcripts, Quarter Sessions, *R v Jagger*.

State Records NSW. 1954. Criminal Transcripts, Quarter Sessions, *R v Sampson*.

State Records NSW. 1958. Criminal Transcripts, Quarter Sessions, *R v Thymes*.

Strong, C. 1932. Public Record Office Victoria, Capital Case Files, Letter to Attorney General from Charles Strong, VPRS 264/P0001/10.

Tasmania. 1921. *The Indeterminate Sentences Act* https://www.austlii.edu.au/cgi-bin/viewdb/au/legis/tas/num_act/tisa192112gvn44342/. Accessed on 18 September 2024.

Victoria. 1944. *Report of the Director of Mental Hygiene*. Melbourne: Government Printer.

Victoria. 1948. *Statute Law Revision Committee on the Crime Bill*. Melbourne: Government Printer.

Who Killed Chrissie Venn? *Advocate*, August 27 1921. http://nla.gov.au/nla.news-article66548914. Accessed on 18 September 2024.

Would Act as Hangman. *Western Star and Roma Advertiser*, 24 September 1932. http://nla.gov.au/nla.news-article98141090. Accessed on 18 September 2024.

## Secondary Material

Angelides, Steven. 2005. The Emergence of the Paedophile in the Late Twentieth Century. *Australian Historical Studies* 36: 272–295. https://doi.org/10.1080/10314610508682924.

Basannavar, Nicholas Ranjan Gadsby. 2018. Speaking About Speaking About Child Sexual Abuse in Britain, 1965–1991. Unpublished PhD thesis, Birkbeck, University of London.

Bashford, Alison, and Carolyn Strange. 2003. *Isolation: Places and Practices of Exclusion*. London: Routledge.

Baynton, Douglas C. 2016. *Defectives in the Land: Disability and Immigration in the Age of Eugenics*. Chicago: The University of Chicago Press.

Blakemore, Tamara, James Leslie Herbert, Fiona Arney, and Samantha Parkinson. 2017. The Impacts of Institutional Child Sexual Abuse: A Rapid Review of the Evidence. *Child Abuse & Neglect* 74: 35–48. https://doi.org/10.1016/j.chiabu.2017.08.006.

Blewer, Robyn. 2021. *Child Witnesses in Twentieth Century Australian Courtrooms*. Cham: Springer International Publishing. https://doi.org/10.1007/978-3-030-69791-4.

Boxall, Hayley, Adam M. Tomison, and Shann Hulme. 2014. *Historical Review of Sexual Offence and Child Sexual Abuse Legislation in Australia: 1788–2013*. Canberra: Australian Institute of Criminology.

Chauncey, George. 1993. The Postwar Sex Crime Panic. In *True Stories From American Past*, ed. W. Graebner, 160–178. New York: McGraw-Hill.

Chenier, Elise. 2003. The Criminal Sexual Psychopath in Canada: Sex, Psychiatry and the Law at Mid- Century. *Canadian Bulletin of Medical History* 20: 75–101.

Durnian, Lisa. 2021. Containing the Undesirables: Discretion and the Sentencing of Habitual Criminals in Australian Supreme Courts in the Twentieth Century. In *History & Crime,* ed. T.J. Kehoe and J.E. Pfeifer, 77–96. Leeds: Emerald Publishing Limited. https://doi.org/10.1108/978-1-80117-698-920211006.

Evans, Carolyn. 2017. Idealists, Pragmatists and 'Simple-Minded' Scamps: The Tasmanian Mental Deficiency Board and State 'Care' in the 1920s. *Australian Historical Studies* 48: 264–279. https://doi.org/10.1080/1031461X.2017.1279195.

Evans, Carolyn, and Naomi Parry. 2001. Vessels of Progressivism? Tasmanian State Girls and Eugenics, 1900–1940. *Australian Historical Studies* 32: 322–333. https://doi.org/10.1080/10314610108596168.

Featherstone, Lisa. 2011. *Let's Talk About Sex: Histories of Sexuality in Australia from Federation to the Pill.* Cambridge: Cambridge Scholars Publishing.

Featherstone, Lisa, and Andy Kaladelfos. 2016. *Sex Crimes in the Fifties.* Melbourne: Melbourne University Press.

Featherstone, Lisa. 2017. The Science of Pleasure: Medicine and Sex Therapy in Mid-twentieth-century Australia. *Social History of Medicine* 31: 446–461.

Featherstone, Lisa. 2018. 'Children in a Terrible State': Understandings of Trauma and Child Sexual Assault in 1970s and 1980s Australia. *Journal of Australian Studies* 42: 164–176.

Find & Connect Web Resource Project (ND). Gosford Training School - Organisation - Find & Connect - New South Wales https://www.findandconnect.gov.au/ref/nsw/biogs/NE01149b.htm. Accessed on 25 March 2024.

Finnane, Mark, Andy Kaladelfos, Alana Piper, Yorick Smaal, Robyn Blewer, and Lisa Durnian, Lisa, et al. 2023. *The Prosecution Project Database [PP]* https://prosecutionproject.griffith.edu.au/prosecutions (version 1, 1 December 2023).

Freedman, Estelle B. 1989. 'Uncontrolled desires': The Response to the Sexual Psychopath, 1920–1960. In *Passion and Power: Sexuality in History*, ed. K. Peiss and C. Simmons, 199–225. Philadelphia: Temple University Press.

Garton, Stephen. 2010. Eugenics in Australia and New Zealand: Laboratories of Race Science. In *InThe Oxford Handbook of Eugenics*, ed. A. Bashford and P. Levine, 243–257. Oxford: Oxford University Press.

Hailes, Helen P., Rongqin Yu, Andrea Danese and Seena Fazel. 2019. Long-Term Outcomes of Childhood Sexual Abuse: An Umbrella Review. *The Lancet Psychiatry* 6: 830–39. https://doi.org/10.1016/S2215-0366(19)30286-X.

Kaladelfos, Andy. 2012. The Politics of Punishment: Rape and the Death Penalty in Colonial Australia, 1841–1901. *History Australia* 9: 155–175.

Kaladelfos, Andy, and Lisa Featherstone. 2016. Sexual Assault by Teachers: Historical Legislative, Policy, and Prosecutorial Responses. In *The Sexual Abuse of Children: Recognition and Redress*, ed. Y. Smaal, A. Kaladelfos, and M. Finnane, 20–34. Clayton: Monash University Publishing.

Kaladelfos, Andy. 2019. Uncovering a Hidden Offence: Social and Legal Histories of Familial Sexual Abuse. In *Gender Violence in Australia: Historical Perspectives*, ed. A. Stevenson and A. Piper, 63–77. Clayton: Monash University Publishing.

Andy, Kaladelfos, and Alana Jayne Piper. 2022. Criminal Justice After the Convicts: A History of the Long Twentieth Century. In *Cambridge Legal History of Australia*, ed. P. Cane, L. Ford, and M. Macmillan, 605–628. Cambridge: Cambridge University Press.

Lira, Natalie. 2021. *Laboratory of Deficiency: Sterilization and Confinement in California, 1900–1950s*. Berkeley: University of California Press.

Lussier, Patrick, Evan C. McCuish, and Jesse Cale. 2021. *Understanding Sexual Offending: An Evidence-Based Response to Myths and Misconceptions*. Cham: Springer International Publishing. https://doi.org/10.1007/978-3-030-53301-4.

McAlinden, Anne Marie. 2014. Deconstructing Victim and Offender Identities in Discourses on Child Sexual Abuse: Hierarchies, Blame and the Good/Evil Dialectic. *The British Journal of Criminology* 54: 180–198. https://doi.org/10.1093/bjc/azt070.

McGregor, Russel. 2002. 'Breed out the Colour' or the Importance of Being White. *Australian Historical Studies* 33: 286–302. https://doi.org/10.1080/10314610208596220.

Petrow, Stefan. 1995. The Furies of Hobart: Women and the Tasmanian Criminal Law in the Early Twentieth Century. *Australian Journal of Law and Society* 11: 67–90.

Smithers, Kathryn. 2023. Contemporary Constructions of 'Sex Offenders'. Unpublished PhD thesis, University of New South Wales.

Strange, Carolyn. 2018. Determining the Punishment of Sex Criminals in Confederation-Era Canada: A Matter of National Policy. *The Canadian Historical Review* 99: 541–562.

Strange, Carolyn. 2020. *The Death Penalty and Sex Murder in Canadian History*. Toronto: Osgoode Society for Canadian Legal History.

Terry, Karren. 2007. Sexual Predators: Diversion, Civil Commitment, Community Reintegration, Challenges, and Opportunities. In *Public Health Behind Bars: From Prisons to Communities*, ed. R.B. Greifinger, 478–492. New York: Springer. https://doi.org/10.1007/978-0-387-71695-4_27.

Wilson, Ron. 2014. Joseph Akeroyd: Rediscovering a Prison Reformer. Unpublished PhD thesis, RMIT University.

# Challenging Ideas of 'Vulnerability' in Prevention of Violence Through the Stories, Experiences and Advocacy of Women with Disabilities

*Patsie Frawley*

## 1 Introduction

> There is this cascading devaluing, discounting that just picks up and grows with momentum to the point where when we hear about the abuse of a woman with a disability, we don't turn to the same sorts of answers around that or ways of describing and understanding it. We go straight to ideas of problem, vulnerable, it's your difference that made this happen. (Patsie Frawley, Disability Royal Commission, transcript 13.10.21)
>
> We will make little progress until we recognise ableism and the intersecting forms of inequality and discrimination that are the underlying drivers of violence and abuse of women and girls with disability. (Commonwealth of Australia 2023)

P. Frawley (✉)
National Centre of Excellence in Intellectual Disability Health, University of New South Wales, Sydney, Australia
e-mail: patsie.frawley@unsw.edu.au





R. E. Keyse et al. (eds.), *Sexual Violence in Medicine and Psychiatry*, Genders and Sexualities in History,
https://doi.org/10.1007/978-3-032-10800-5_5

Prevention of sexual violence against women and girls with disabilities needs to be a part of broader gender-based violence prevention efforts. Prevention of violence against women is internationally understood as a social systemic approach that uses an analysis of gender-based power. The Equality Institute and UN Women define primary prevention of gender-based violence as 'Policy and programme initiatives aimed at addressing the underlying causes and factors of violence against women and girls including systems, structures, norms, attitudes, practices, and power imbalances' (The Equality Institute and UN Women 2023. 4). This definition aligns with an ecological model of gender-based violence and abuse that is used by these agencies and the World Health Organisation (see Fig. 1) that nests individual, relational, community and societal factors as impacting on experiences of violence and as sites of prevention, with the broadest level or macro level being societal.

This model positions violence against women as a social problem that requires social transformation to prevent all forms of violence. Violence against women in this way is seen as an ecology of inter-related socially constructed factors, and violence prevention presented as an ecological model requiring work at each level. The WHO notes that the model reinforces that 'no single factor can explain why some people or groups are at higher risk of interpersonal violence' (World Health Organisation n.d.). However, for women with disabilities the single factor of disability is commonly applied when considering violence against them. Tethered to

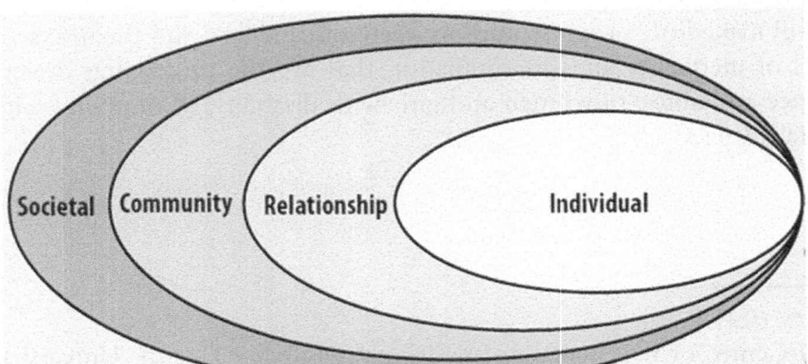


**Fig. 1** The ecological model Krug, G. E., Dahlberg, L., Mercy, J. A., Zwi, A. B., & Lozano, R. (2002). World report on health and violence (p. 12). World Health Organization

this understanding of disability is the often uncontested idea that women with disabilities are inherently vulnerable.

In this chapter, research that has used the stories of women with disabilities who have experienced violence and abuse and an ecological analysis of these experiences is presented to challenge the 'inherently vulnerable' narrative of women with disabilities that have framed policy and practice. It explores how a systemic understanding of prevention of violence and abuse can be framed through these stories and the adoption of an ecological model that considers the intersecting social and systemic factors that have shaped women with disabilities' experiences.

## 2 Disability Violence and Abuse

Like gender, disability has been used as a single reason for violence and abuse. Notions of the inherent vulnerability of people with disabilities have shaped legislation, policy and practice that led to the systemic segregation, institutionalisation and isolation of people with disabilities away from and outside of society. These responses to disability ultimately set up systems and practices where violence, abuse, neglect and exploitation have been prevalent, and occurring outside the public gaze. The irony is, service models that came from these responses, including special schools, residential institutions often run by religious orders, sheltered employment and segregated congregate residential services were understood socially as being protective for disabled people.

### *2.1 Vulnerability and Disability*

Canadian disability researcher Dick Sobsey undertook research about violence and abuse experienced by people with disabilities to 're-frame' the understanding of the 'causes' of abuse from an individual to a systemic framing. His work from the mid-1990s began a change in focus on disability violence and abuse that is reflected in the work of current researchers and the Royal Commissions of Inquiry outlined later in the chapter. This research and advocacy stresses 'that society's response to disability may be more important than the disability itself in increasing vulnerability and may imply that intervention must be aimed primarily at systems rather than individuals' (Sobsey 2004, 99). Other researchers have drawn on Sobsey's work to further develop and apply the ecological model of disability violence and abuse to prevention policy, training and programmes (Frawley and O'Shea 2019; Fitzsimons 2009; Hollomotz 2009). A characteristic of this work is advocacy for social change that positions people with disabilities as change agents through being co-researchers, co-producers of prevention approaches and co-facilitators of prevention programmes, acknowledging their capacity and agency, and hearing and using their voices to question the ableist systems that have positioned them as vulnerable.

Before Sobsey's work, the increased risk of sexual violence and abuse experienced by people with developmental and intellectual disabilities was seen to be caused by the perceived dependency and cognitive incapacity of people with disability. This idea of dependency extended to beliefs about incapacity to give informed consent to sexual and romantic engagement; they could not think or act independently. The dominant narrative was therefore they could not 'know the difference' between consensual and abusive sex, and did not have the 'mental capacity' or agency to make decisions about sex and sexual relationships. This deficit focus has underpinned much of the academic, public and in some cases legal discourse on disability violence and abuse for decades. While aligning strongly with the medical and charity models of disability (Clifton 2020) the discourse and the practices it has informed remain in circulation today in many countries. A recent example is the media reporting on the rape and murder of Lena Zhang Harrap in Auckland New Zealand in 2023:

> Her physical impairments, the combination with her diagnosis of Down Syndrome, and the associated impairments that came with that, placed her in a degree of vulnerability that was not seen in a number of comparable cases presented to the court. (Blackwell and Forman, RNZ, 4 May 2023)

Here vulnerability is firmly placed 'within' Lena rather than looking at the engrained gendered nature of violence, sexual abuse, rape and in this case murder.

### 2.2 *Challenging the Status 'Vulnerable'*

Victim blaming like that referred to above resonates with decades of examples where characteristics of female gender have been referred to in similar ways to 'explain' acts of sexual and other violence against women. The discourse here is about vulnerability of women or within women and even further a discourse of 'blame for' the sexual violence and abuse they experience. To some extent this narrative has shifted in relation to gender based violence in the public domain through grass roots movements like #MeToo. However, the kind of reporting reflected in relation to the rape and murder of Lena Zhang Harrap strongly suggests there is a long way to go to challenge the hard wired views that to be disabled, and to be a disabled woman in particular equates to being vulnerable to sexual abuse and other forms of violence because of the presumed deficits of the person. In Australia and New Zealand two government inquiries have explored experiences of violence and abuse of people with disabilities in ways that challenge the presumed deficit perspective, thereby offering a challenge to the idea of inherent vulnerability of people with disabilities.

The recent Australian *Royal Commission into Violence, Abuse, Neglect and Exploitation of People with Disabilities* 2019–2023 clearly records that these models of education, housing and employment were places of abuse and human rights violations. Importantly the 222 recommendations of this Royal Commission repeat the need to radically change and deconstruct these systems through a human rights approach. The report notes,

> They [the named commissioners] consider the segregation of people with disability, including in education, to be a significant human rights issue linked with violence against, and the abuse, neglect and exploitation of, people with disability. (Commonwealth of Australia 2023, 79)

The scope of the Royal Commission and its approach were framed by an ecological model of disability violence as it conducted hearings with a focus on key parts of the system—education, health, housing, and it engaged in questioning that were focussed using individual stories (evidence) within the context of relationships (family, services) and within the context of community, and society (government policy). The inquiry was also clearly informed by a human rights model of disability with particular reference to the United Nations Convention on the Rights of Persons with Disabilities (UN 2006). Importantly the Australian Royal Commission also noted the need for an intersectional understanding of disability violence and abuse, with a particular focus on intersections of gender and culture. This shaped a broad inquiry that has developed far reaching recommendations for social change that are based on an unequivocal respect for the personhood of people with disabilities and is a clear example of the systemic understanding of violence and abuse and its prevention in practice.

In a similar way, the *New Zealand Royal Commision of Inquiry into Abuse in Care 2021–2024*, a broader inquiry that focuses on State and Faith-based care from the 1950s through to 1999, notes, 'many children and young persons from all communities were removed from their families and placed in care' (Commonwealth of New Zealand 2018, 18), recognises the intersecting factors impacting experiences of violence and abuse. In this inquiry these include; culture in particular Māori and Pacific cultures, age, in particular youth and young people, disability and mental illness. This inquiry has also taken a systemic approach in particular noting the increased risk of abuse inherent within the segregated institutions that were a part of the state and faith-based care, that are recognised as closed systems dominated by colonial and welfare paradigms.

Research undertaken with people with intellectual disabilities for the New Zealand inquiry used an ecological model of disability violence and abuse to analyse and understand the individual, relational, community and societal factors impacting on the lives of people with disabilities who experienced abuse in care, and how these factors including colonialism and ableism, created environments where the violence and abuse could occur—again seemingly outside of the public gaze (Mirfin-Veitch et al. 2022). The analysis of the stories of people with intellectual disability aimed to position the individual stories of violence and abuse shared in the research, within the broader social contexts where and when the abuse experienced took place.

The report highlights how the systems put in place by the State to support and protect children and young people failed them—repeatedly and catastrophically—constituting systemic abuse. (Abuse in Care Royal Commission of Inquiry n.d.).

As the two inquiries referred to in this chapter evidence, systemic abuse of people with disabilities has grown from ideas of vulnerability at the individual level of disability. This individually focused, inherently vulnerable discourse, has dominated practices worldwide; particularly for women with disabilities, and particularly for women with intellectual disabilities. This has played out most starkly in the area of sexuality and relationships where myths and stereotypes about the vulnerability of women with intellectual disabilities have restricted their right to be sexual, to claim their sexual identity and to self-determine the way they want to express their sexuality. Some of these myths include that women with disabilities are asexual, hypersexual, unable to or incapable of consent and not intimate, sexual people (Azzopardi-Lane and Callus 2015; Fitzgerald and Withers 2011; McCarthy 2014; O'Shea and Frawley 2020). Again, practices put in place to 'protect' women with intellectual disabilities including sterilisation, congregate care and institutionalisation have instead been places and practices of abuse.

An individual, deficit or impairment analysis of vulnerability does not fit with the current theoretical and advocacy analysis and understanding of disability which has been shaped by the social model of disability, and disability activism through the voices of people with disabilities since at least the 1970s (Huemann and Joiner 2020). Gains made by this work have resulted in a shift towards a rights-based model of disability enshrined in the United Nations Convention on the Rights of Persons with Disabilities (CRPD) which has at its centre the equal legal and personhood status of people with disabilities. Article 3 (a) notes a key principle of the CRPD is 'Respect for inherent dignity, individual autonomy including the freedom to make one's own choices, and independence of persons' (United Nations 2006). While the CRPD has supported some legislative reform, and progressive policy and practice in areas of inclusive education, fair and equal employment, accessible health including women's health and sexual health, and legislation for reproductive rights, these gains have been to a greater or lesser extent dependant on societal level factors including domestic government disability policy, and local level practices of disability support.

### 2.3 *Challenging Ideas of Safeguarding 'The Vulnerable'*

Countries that have signed and ratified the CRPD have begun legislative reform about decision making rights, and restrictive decision making practice using Article 12 of the CRPD which has a focus on legal capacity and decision making (O'Mahony and de Paor 2023; O'Mahony 2023; Domanski and Lackoronski 2023). This work has engaged with questions of capacity, and balancing support and safeguarding measures that might restrict decision making. Article 12 (4) notes that any safeguards to prevent abuse must 'respect the rights, will and preferences of the person..[and be] proportional to the degree to which the measures affect the person's rights and interests'.

In the area of disability violence and abuse prevention there is still much work to do to gain the balance between autonomy/agency and protection/risk mitigation, particularly for women with intellectual disabilities and others for whom cognitive and mental/emotional interaction with the world is challenging. For them often the pendulum swings further to protective and restrictive approaches regarding their decision making about relationships and sexuality based on ideas of 'inherent vulnerability'. While Australian and New Zealand jurisdictions do not have the same legal basis for 'Adult Safeguarding' as the UK, it is interesting that in these countries there is a strong focus on 'safeguarding' people with intellectual and other cognitive disabilities in practice. This is most evident when hearing the stories of people who have experienced these restrictions, as reflected in the stories in the later part of this chapter. Laura Pritchard-Jones in their critique of UK practices of safeguarding notes that a 'status-based' label of vulnerability is often applied to these groups (Pritchard-Jones 2018), and this approach has led to what they say have been 'poorly defined responses' to perceived vulnerability or 'risk'.

### 2.4 *Intersections of Gender, Disability and Violence and Abuse*

The CRPD recognises the intersections of gender, disability and abuse in Article 6 that notes that 'states Parties recognise that women and girls with disabilities are subject to multiple discriminations' that increase risk to violence and abuse. Stienstra (2023) in their analysis of gender, disability and disability rights in transnational and international relations points out.

The acknowledged situation is that women and girls with disabilities are among the most excluded, marginalised, or disadvantaged women or people in the world and experience intersectional discrimination which increases their barriers and limits their ability to claim their rights. (Stienstra 2023, 355)

One of these rights is the right to safety as articulated in the CRPD. Statistics reporting violence and abuse against women with disabilities reflects the way in which intersectional discrimination has impacted on this right. In Australia it is reported by the Australian Bureau of Statistics, that young women with disabilities are twice as likely as young women without disabilities to experience sexual violence (9% compared to 4%) (Centre of Research Excellence in Disability and Health n.d.). Research based on the 2019 New Zealand Family Violence Study reported that forty percent of disabled women experience physical violence from an intimate partner over their lifetimes, compared with twenty-five per cent of non-disabled women (Fanslow et al 2021). In the UK the Disability and Crime, 2019 report found that in

> the three years ending March 2018, disabled women were almost twice as likely to have experienced any sexual assault in the last year (5.7%) than non-disabled women (3.0%) and disabled women were more than twice as likely to have experienced domestic abuse (17.3%) than non-disabled women (7.%). (Office of National Statistics 2019)

While these high rates of violence and abuse continue to be reported there is a need to ask how prevention of violence can be achieved.

The ecological model of disability violence and abuse first proposed by Sobsey has played a very important part in shifting the gaze from the individual and their disability to a more systemic understanding of disability violence and abuse. It also aligns clearly with mainstream ecological models of violence and abuse enabling important cross disciplinary and cross sector work as evidenced by programmes like 'Sexual Lives and Respectful Relationships' outlined later in the chapter (Frawley and O'Shea 2019). Increasingly the model has also opened up opportunities to understand disability violence and abuse from an intersectional perspective, as outlined earlier through references to current and recent inquiries into disability violence and abuse. The next step in the evolution of this model might be to consider what a comprehensive ecological model of gendered ableist violence and abuse could look like and how such a model could be used to advocate for the positioning of women with disabilities as advocates for change. It is the aim of the remainder of this chapter to show how the stories of women with disabilities, and the centring of their stories and experiences in programmes that aim to prevent violence are the powerful tools needed.

It is this possibility that informed the narrative research and prevention and advocacy work associated with the research that is described and drawn on in the remainder of the chapter; Sexual Lives and Respectful Relationships—an Australian body of work spanning fifteen years that used narrative research to co-develop a sexuality rights programme with women with intellectual disabilities (Frawley and O'Shea 2019; Frawley 2023), Mean As!—a New Zealand study using a co-researching method with people with intellectual disabilities to co-develop, analyse and produce stories and resources to inform a sexuality rights understanding of disability and sexuality (Luskie et al. 2019; Milner et al 2019), and 'Tell me About You' (Mirfin-Veitch et al. 2022) research undertaken to inform the hearings about people with intellectual disabilities at the New Zealand Royal Inquiry into Abuse in State Care which also gathered and analysed stories with people with disabilities about their experiences of abuse.

The following section aims to share the stories of a number of women with disabilities who have experienced violence and abuse and to reflect on how these stories have been and can continue to shape and frame prevention of violence efforts.

## 3 Women with Disabilities' 'Own and Owned' Stories

Mean As! is an online library of stories that were co-developed with people with intellectual disabilities[1] in New Zealand to tell the stories of relationship and sexuality experiences. The aim was to hear previously unheard voices to inform a rights approach to an area which had for decades been either silenced or dominated by professional-led research and practice. The website of Mean As! notes

> Although a lot has been written about the relational and sexual lives of people with a learning disability, very little has been written by them. In the absence of stories that are recognisably their own, we have come to know people with a learning disability and what they can and can't do, from the story telling of those who exercise power over them. People with a learning disability tell us that this silence has meant they are routinely prevented from talking about, learning about and ultimately enjoying the same sexual rights as every other citizen. (Donald Beasley Institute 2019)

Three of the seven stories include the voices and experiences of women with an intellectual disability. The research project was co-designed and undertaken by a research group including two women with intellectual disabilities. The research group had five guiding questions: 1. How the story made us feel; 2. What we thought the Storyteller was trying to tell us; 3.Why their story was important to them and why it was important for others to hear; 4. Why they might have told their story that way and why they have made the decisions they did; and 5. What needed to change

[1] Note the term 'Learning Disability' is used in NZ.

if people with a learning disability were going to tell better stories in the future (Donald Beasley Institute 2019). Two reports were developed from the study (Milner et al. 2019; Luskie et al. 2019) and the online library remains an active part of the research centre's research focus. The research group noted that one outcome they wanted from the work was, 'we thought we had created an opportunity for people to talk to each other about the stories and whether what happened to the Storytellers was fair. That is why we have libraries after all!' (Luskie et al. 2019).

### *3.1 Sexual Lives and Respectful Relationships*

This program, or as some refer to it 'movement' was developed from work undertaken in the early 2000s at the Australian Research Centre in Sex, Health and Society at LaTrobe University Melbourne. This research, *Living Safer Sexual Lives (LSSL)* aimed to gather the life stories of people with intellectual disability with a focus on sexuality and relationships to better understand how sexuality had been managed in their lives, and how sexuality rights had been engaged with by people with intellectual disabilities (Johnson et al. 2002). The research informed the development of a training programme that included the 25 stories and 3 sets of training modules that used the stories as the key learning materials; one set of training for people with intellectual disabilities, one for disability staff and one for families (Frawley et al. 2004). This approach was used to reflect the ecological model of disability violence and abuse referred to earlier developed by Dick Sobsey; it recognised that if violence and abuse were to be prevented changes were needed at the individual, relational, community and societal/systems levels. The training programme ran across Australia, New Zealand and internationally. Leading on from this work the *Sexual Lives and Respectful Relationships* (SL&RR) programme was developed using a number of the stories from LSSL and adding a peer education model that engaged people with intellectual disabilities as co-facilitators of the programme with community professionals in sexuality, sexual health and sexual assault services (Deakin University n.d.).

Central to this work are the stories of people with an intellectual disability from LSSL, adding new stories over the decade of this program's work to include stories by LGBTQ people with intellectual disabilities (Marks et al. 2020) and young people with intellectual disability (Frawley 2023; Deakin University n.d.). These stories and this model of prevention are synonymous with disability violence and abuse prevention work in Australia and remain in use in a key regional programme in the state of Victoria where it has been operating for over ten years. The programme is co-led by a disability self-advocacy group and a regional sexual assault service where SL&RR is funded and embedded in their prevention work.

### 3.2 *Tell Me About You: A Life Story Approach to Understanding Disabled People's Experiences in Care (1950–1999)*

This research was undertaken as part of the New Zealand Royal Commision of Inquiry into State Care (Abuse in Care Royal Commission of Inquiry n.d.) to '...provide people with learning disabilities and neurodiversity an opportunity to share their experiences from State and faith-based care, and have their voices heard' (Mirfin-Veitch et al. 2022, 8). In all, 16 people told their stories with researchers from the DBI; 12 were male and four were female. The stories were presented within a report that included an ecological analysis to explore and understand '...the interrelatedness of factors that both impact on disabled people, and create environments where violence and abuse is able to occur' (Mirfin-Veitch et al. 2022, 12). The stories of abuse told by the people who engaged with this project were also presented as evidence at a contextual hearing of the Royal Inquiry into abuse in State Care that focussed on experiences of people with disabilities (Royal Commission of Inquiry—Abuse in Care n.d.). In the media reports from this hearing Dr Brigit Mirfin-Veitch the director of the DBI who presented the findings of the report noted, 'Survivors also experienced sexual violence that was an "inescapable and unchallenged reality" for disabled people[2] in care' (Scotcher 2019).

### 3.3 *'Told stories'—Challenging Ideas of Vulnerability*

These three projects have 'given voice' to the experiences of more than fifty people with disabilities about their lives. An overview of these stories also tells a history of violence and abuse that runs through the life experiences as told by people for whom 'being heard' has not been part of these experiences. This section shares some excerpts from the stories and the key messages they provide that challenge dominant ideas about what makes a woman with an intellectual disability vulnerable to sexual violence

[2] 'Disabled People' is the preferred term used in New Zealand. This was advocated for and determined by the disability community.

challenging 'individually' focused, vulnerability framed understandings of disability violence and abuse.

### 3.3.1 *Lusi (Lusi is Non Verbal and Now Uses a Communication Aide to Communicate. This Storyteller Chose to Use Their Real Name)*

During the day, we sat in the recreational room but there were no activities ... we hardly interacted with each other... The institute felt 'dark and cold' ... I did not know how to express myself. There were no tools or strategies offered to me to communicate with people around me—so I could express what I wanted and needed... No one thought to ask me what was going on for me... No one ever talked to me about my Samoan heritage either. ... There was no respect or effort to recognise me for who I am...Returning to live with mum was challenging. She was in an abusive relationship... we had to escape from mum's boyfriend eventually... We went to the women's refuge first... There was no freedom of choice in entering care. I was lost in care (Mirfin-Veitch et al. 2022).

Lusi's story, told in part here, tells of the pervasiveness of abuse in her life firstly through the institution she was placed in, later at the hands of an abusive man who was her mother's partner, and later again within the community care system. In the institution she was given no way of expressing herself and was therefore left to have no social interactions and no emotional safety. Looking at the ways in which violence and abuse framed Lusi's life it is difficult to look past the systemic context. Choices were made about her placement, her communication and her identity that paid little to no attention to who she was, including culturally. Lusi reminds us that it is freedom not protection that she needed to 'live her life her way'.

### 3.3.2 *Gina (Not the Storyteller's Real Name)*

My stepfather abused me... If my mother wouldn't give him sex, he'd turn to me or my older sister... Mum'd have guys over and sleep with them... Sex was just like that... One day I ran away. My older sister's husband came into the caravan and raped me, and that was my last option. When I left home that day I went on a swing and I stayed on the swing all day saying, 'I'm a good girl, I'm not a bad girl, I'm a good girl, I'm a good girl.'... An old copper found me and took me to the cop station. They took me back to my mum's house. I was scared. I was like a crushed leaf. The police woman was holding me up. My mum said, 'We don't know her, we don't want her in this house. Take her away.'... (Johnson et al. 2001).

Earlier in Gina's story she talks about being treated differently than her siblings, not getting the food and love they got, and her siblings and her mother sexually and physically abusing her. Gina experienced extreme violence and abuse 'because of her disability' in a family that punished her for her difference/her disability. The sexual violence experienced and told in Gina's full story was too hard for the Sexual Lives and Respectful Relationships peer educators to work with. As a team the women peer educators chose to remove Gina's story from the SL&RR programme. I remember the discussions clearly and the difficulty of those discussions; these women were also Gina's peers—they did not know her but through her story they connected and expressed the need to 'care for Gina'. They did not feel they could do that by presenting her story 'on her behalf', nor did they feel they could look after their safety and the safety of other women with disabilities who, like Gina, experienced extreme violence, abuse and abandonment by their families. The women peer educators' camaraderie and advocacy through their actions to keep Gina safe by keeping her story safe were a clear reflection of their understanding of the enduring impact of family violence against people with disabilities.

The relational context of Gina's story of violence and abuse is an important reminder that when looking at reasons for risk of violence and abuse against people with disabilities, the 'value' or 'devaluing' of the person within their family units can be where the vulnerability is shaped. However, for Gina she did not feel vulnerable to violence and abuse once she was in a 'safe place', which for her was disability supported accommodation. Her reflection that 'she never looked back' is an important message about the strength and resilience of women with disabilities when they have the right environment to express it.

Gina's story concludes with her sharing her reflections on her love for her partner Cathy and for women.

> Cathy and I were made for each other. She looks after me. I can't read and write very well and she helps me. She has been there from the start. She is always there for me. Loving a woman is like loving everything you want in life. I've never liked a man in my whole life. I think to me loving a woman is like loving yourself. Women have a lot more than men. Honesty, open and caring. And their bodies! Oh yeah their bodies! (Johnson et al. 2001, 12).

### 3.3.3 *Sometimes I Write Letters (This Storyteller Chose Not to Use a Name—Just the Title of Their Story)*

...I want to let you know that my story talks about hard things, but they are things that are important to say. I am not impressed with what happened with me, nor am I happy with the actions of my rapists. It has made me very upset and angry. My abusers took advantage of me when I was a child and I lost my innocence because of it... I remember, on one occasion, I had gone over to the netball courts and was playing with one of my sisters and a friend. I felt thirsty so I went to get a drink of water. That's when he came up to me and told me we were going for a walk. We went for a long walk through the school...He then attacked me, making my friend (who he had also taken with us) watch while he raped me... (Luskie et al. 2019, 39).

This storyteller's story reads like the script that supports the individually focussed discourse of disability and vulnerability covered earlier in this chapter—people with intellectual disabilities do not know how to protect themselves, they are not 'capable' of understanding danger, they are 'inherently vulnerable'. However, in this story the storyteller reflects their innocence—she was a child at the time, like many children she obeyed an older person and she had no idea that a walk would lead to rape. This is more like other stories of child sexual abuse than different from it. If we see the 'child' first and not the disability does it read any differently? The storyteller, an adult when they told their story reflects a strong 'survivor' narrative. Running throughout the full story is a list of recommendations for others who experience abuse.

> I want you to know that abuse is not your fault and you don't deserve all the pain and hurt. But I know it makes you wonder why me? This can make you feel sick, angry, hurt, lonely, trapped, stuck, unloved and unappreciated. I want you to carry on, keep loving yourself and get good sleep! (Luski et al. 2019, 40)

This story was a favourite of the Mean As! research group of disabled people who worked with these stories to develop a set of 'key messages' to share alongside the stories in the online library including

> Even though the Storyteller was writing about rape and the impact that it had had on her life, we felt the story was a letter of hope, especially to people who had been sexually assaulted.

> This story is important to hear because it is the story of a woman with a learning disability – and not someone else. We are the experts in our own lives. This letter has important messages for people with a learning disability who have been abused. Most especially that abuse is not your fault. Abuse is about the person doing it – not the person who has been abused. (Luskie et al. 2019, 40 – 41)

### 3.3.4 *Aliyah's Story (Aliyah is Not the Storyteller's Real Name. It is a Story Co-developed in an SL&RR Project with Young People with Disabilities)*

> I left home in a taxi and went to a shelter. I remember in the back seat of the Taxi, feeling sad and down, thinking why was I put in the situation of needing to leave home? Was it because I needed to 'save' my own life from continuing to be abused? Or was it because I needed to have somewhere safe to live? Who knows?
> I lived in homeless shelters for a few months. It gave me some time to get my life together and I live in my own unit now. There was something that happened to me at school. I didn't want it to happen... When I went to get help from authorities, I felt like they didn't believe me. I did not consent for the abuse to happen...I spoke up because I didn't want anyone else to be abused and left traumatised like me.. (SL&RR n.d)

Aliyah's story is a story of hard-won independence and recovery. The abuse they experienced was at a school and was perpetrated by someone employed at the school—a person in a position of power over Aliyah. Aliyah tells of not being believed and having to seek out support for their story to be heard, if not believed, elsewhere. The staff member being stood down appears to be the only acknowledgement of the abuse. Again a too common story of systems like education having a closed approach to reporting of abuse. The inquiries into abuse referred to earlier have countless tellings of similar stories of abuse in education and other services for people with disabilities where the system 'sweeps it under the carpet'. Aliyah does not talk about the perpetrator of the abuse in detail but tells us the important piece of information about them—they were a staff member of the school. Again, the inquiries referred to in this chapter make it clear that people employed to work with people with disabilities are often the perpetrators of abuse. This is well documented in cases including the Yooralla cases in Victoria Australia where staff members were found guilty of abuse of people with disabilities in residential services,[3] and the Winterbourne cases in the UK where six staff were jailed for abusing residents in a disability care home.[4] In these cases the exposure of the abuse was by whistleblowers who in one of the Yooralla cases and the Winterbourne case used hidden cameras to reveal the abuse, and the media to publicly expose the abuse. Aliyah did not have these tools or people to help her expose her abuse.

The need for safety is central to Aliyah's story—safety 'at home', safety in relationships, cultural safety. For Aliyah independence 'from' family and services provided this safety. If thinking about Aliyah's experiences of abuse and their survival and reclaiming of their agency using an ecological model, we can see again that factors at the systems and societal level have been impactful—gender, culture, disability and at the relational level—family. These intersect in ways that have been abusive, enabled abuse and been sites of abuse. At the centre of the experiences—the individual level, is a strong young woman whose striving for independence has positioned her as able, capable and valued and an advocate for her rights and the rights of others in her cultural and disability communities.

### *3.4 Sexuality and Relationship Rights*

In the early 2000s Ann Craft, a disability researcher from the UK, wrote about sexuality in the lives of people with intellectual disabilities using a rights framework. In this work Craft articulated a set of sexual rights that she argued were a more positive way to begin to think about sexuality in the lives of people with intellectual disability—where restrictions and managing risk had been the dominant discourse. The rights Craft articulated were;

[3] See, Butcher, Steve and Mark Russell. 2014. Yooralla Worker Jailed For Sexual Abuse Refused Appeal Request. https://www.theage.com.au/national/victoria/yooralla-worker-jailed-for-sexual-abuse-refused-appeal-request-20140530-3981m.html. Accessed 18 September 2024. See also, Russell, Mark. 2015. Former Yooralla Manager Jailed for Sexual Abuse of Autistic Woman. https://www.theage.com.au/national/victoria/former-yooralla-manager-jailed-for-sexual-abuse-of-autistic-woman-20150629-gi0di1.html. Accessed 18 September 2024.

[4] See, Hill, Amelia. 2012. Winterbourne View Care Staff Jailed for Abusing Residents. The Guardian, 26 October. https://www.theguardian.com/society/2012/oct/26/winterbourne-view-care-staff-jailed. Accessed 18 September 2024.

> To be treated like an adult; To be sexual; To have information about sexual health, sex and relationships; To make your own decisions about relationships; To have privacy and be respected at home; To be safe from violence and abuse; To be able to do these things without other people stopping you. (Craft 2004).

The SL&RR programme embedded these rights into the peer-led workshops. Each workshop focussed on a story from the library of stories that had been developed from LSSL research and SL&RR research over almost two decades. The SL&RR project group employed people with intellectual disabilities as co-researchers to co-develop the workshops, to work as peer educators and as peer educator trainers. At its height there were 9 sites across Australia and more than 40 peer educators, all using the stories, the key messages and activities that had been co-developed throughout the programme. The peer educators were in some ways an extension of the stories—like the people in the stories whose sexuality, identity as sexual, and their rights to be sexual and have relationships had been framed by societal views about (mainly women with) intellectual disabilities. They challenged these ideas through the lists of affirming key messages they found in the stories and shared in the programme.

Linda Stokoe was a founding peer educator in SL&RR and stayed working with the programme for more than five years. Presenting at conferences, running the peer educator training and co-developing the large range of resources that accompanied the programme. In one of these resources called the 'Relationships activity' that uses a set of picture cards with different ways people show their affection in relationships, Linda shares the following messages:

> Sometimes people with disabilities don't have the chance to be in a relationship, or they might not understand relationships because they haven't had the right information before, like when they were at school. This is not good. You can't not tell someone something because you think they don't understand. They might actually want to have a relationship and a family.
>
> Having a relationship means that you have another person to talk to, you can go and do things together, or play games, or cuddle, or make love, or help out around the house together. It's hard being on your own, so it is nice to have someone to spend time with. (SL&RR n.d.)

Linda's advocacy through SL&RR is an important legacy of this work that is continuing to influence violence and abuse prevention work led by people with intellectual disabilities. She related through the stories and the programme her own experiences. While academics were also involved in this work the people who owned it were these peer educators and project workers. The SL&RR research team used the ecological model of prevention of violence (Linda called this the 'onion') to frame our work (see Fig. 2).

In this model peer educators are at the centre, building their capacity and the capacity of other people with disabilities to engage with their rights—to be sexual, to be safe, to determine how they run their sexual lives and relationships. Through this they also acted as change agents—in particular through being positioned as the 'experts by experience' with a legitimate role in prevention work (Frawley 2023).

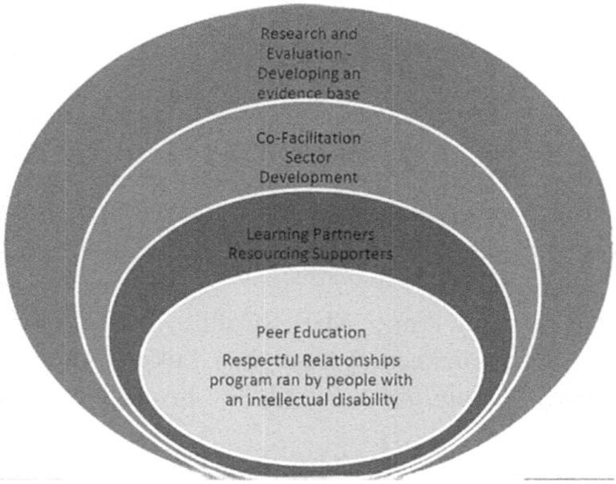


**Fig. 2** The SL&RR model is a translation of Sobsey's ecological model to locate the components of the programme as an ecological prevention of violence programme that centres the work of people with intellectual disabilities as peer educators who are shifting ideas about vulnerability by being experts in their own experiences and using this expertise to work with their peers as educators and as advocates. (author's own work)

## 4 Conclusion

Exploring how vulnerability has been constructed around, and applied to people with disabilities, and in particular women and women with intellectual disabilities has been used as the backdrop to the small insight into the lives of women with disabilities shared here through excerpts of some women's stories. The aim of the chapter was to reflect on, critique and then evidence the problem of a discourse of vulnerability when we are thinking about disability violence and abuse. It is hoped that the work shared in this chapter will lead others to read more stories told by women with disabilities about who they are, how they see themselves and how, despite the gendered ableist and systemic abuse they have experienced they can be and are the voices of change transforming their own and others' lives as rights holders.

**Funding** The author declares no competing interests. No direct funding was received for this work.

## References

Abuse in Care Royal Commission of Inquiry. n.d. https://www.abuseincare.org.nz/our-progress/library/v/528/tell-me-about-you. Accessed on 18 September 2024.

Azzopardi-Lane, Claire, and Anne Marie Callus. 2015. Constructing Sexual Identities: People with Intellectual Disability Talking About Sexuality. *British Journal of Learning Disabilities* 43: 32–37. https://doi.org/10.1111/bld.12083.

Centre of Research Excellence in Disability and Health. n.d. *Melbourne School of Population and Global Health Disability and Health Unit Violence against People with Disability.* Retrieved from https://credh.org.au/nature-and-extent-of-violence/

Clifton, Shane. 2020. Hierarchies of Power: Disability Theories and Models and Their Implications for Violence Against, and Abuse, Neglect, and Exploitation of, People With Disability. *Analysis and Policy Observatory.* https://apo.org.au/node/309065. Accessed on 18 September 2024.

Commonwealth of Australia. 2023. *Royal Commission into Violence, Abuse, Neglect and Exploitation of People with Disability.* Canberra: Commonwealth of Australia.

Commonwealth of New Zealand. 2018. *Terms of Reference - Royal Commission of Inquiry into Historical Abuse in State Care and in the Care of Faith-based Institutions Order 2018*. Wellington, New Zealand: Government of New Zealand.

Craft, Ann. 2004. *Practice Issues in Sexuality and Learning Disabilities*. London: Routledge.

Deakin University. n.d. *Sexual Lives and Respectful Relationships*. https://web.archive.org/web/20220304033436/, https://www.slrr.com.au/research-resources/online-resources/. Accessed on 18 September 2024.

Domanski, Maciej, and Boguslaw Lackoronski. 2023. Comparative Analysis of the Transposition of Article 12 of the UN Convention on the Rights of Persons with Disabilities. In *Models of Implementation of Article 12 of the Convention on the Rights of Persons with Disabilities (CRPD)*, ed. M. Domanski and B. Lackoronski, 600–605. London: Routledge.

Donald Beasley Institute. 2019. *Mean As! People with Learning Disability Telling and Reading Stories of Relationships and Sexuality*. https://www.donaldbeasley.org.nz/projects/mean-as. Accessed on 18 September 2024.

Fanslow, Janet, Zarintaj Malihi, Ladan Hashemi, Pauline Gulliver, and Tracey McIntosh. 2021. Lifetime Prevalence of Intimate Partner Violence and Disability: Results From a Population-based study in New Zealand. *American Journal of Preventive Medicine* 61: 320–328. https://doi.org/10.1016/j.amepre.2021.02.022.

Fitzgerald, Christina, and Paul Withers. 2011. 'I Don't Know What a Proper Woman Means': What Women with Intellectual Disabilities Think About Sex, Sexuality and Themselves. *British Journal of Learning Disabilities* 41: 5–12. https://doi.org/10.1111/j.1468-3156.2011.00715.x.

Fitzsimons, Nancy. 2009. *Combating Violence and Abuse of People with Disabilities: A Call to Action*. Baltimore, MD: Paul H. Brookes.

Frawley, Patsie. 2023. Perspective Chapter: Sexuality and Relationships Education and Advocacy by People with Disabilities Through Peer Education. In *Sexual Education Around the World – Past, Present and Future Issues*. InTechOpen. https://doi.org/10.5772/intechopen.1001318/.

Frawley, Patsie, and Amie O'Shea. 2019. Peer Education: A Platform for Sexuality Rights Advocacy for Women with Intellectual Disabilities. In *Global Perspectives on Disability Activism and Advocacy*, ed. K. Soldatic and K. Johnson. Abingdon: Routledge. https://doi.org/10.4324/9781351237499.

Frawley, Patsie, Kelley Johnson, Lynne Hillier, and Lyn Harrison. 2004. *Living Safer Sexual Lives: A Training and Resource Pack for People with Learning Disabilities and Those Who Support Them*. Brighton: Pavilion Publishing.

Hollomotz, Andrea. 2009. Beyond 'Vulnerability': An Ecological Approach to Conceptualising Risk of Sexual Violence Against People with Learning Difficulties. *British Journal of Social Work* 39: 99–112.

Huemann, Judith, and Kristen Joiner. 2020. *Being Heumann: An Unrepentant Memoir of A Disability Rights Activist*. Boston: Beacon Press.

Johnson, Kelley, Patsie Frawley, Lynne Hillier, and Lyn Harrison. 2002. Living Safer Sexual Lives: Research and Action. *Tizard Learning Disability Review* 7: 4–9.

Johnson, Kelley, Lynne Hillier, Lyn Harrison, and Patsie Frawley. 2001. *Living Safer Sexual Lives - Final Report*. Melbourne: Australian Research Centre in Sex, Health and Society.

Luskie, William., Vanessa Murphy, Darryl White, Cheryl Wallace, Paul Milner, Brigit Mirfin-Veitch, Kelly Tikao, and Patsie Frawley. 2019. *"Mean As!": People with a Learning Disability Telling and Reading Stories of Relationships and Sexuality*. Dunedin, New Zealand: Donald Beasley Institute.

Marks, Genée, Amie O'Shea, Keith R. McVilly, Patsie Frawley, and Nathan Despott. 2020. 'Where's the Human Dignity in That?" LGBTQIA+ People with Intellectual Disability Exploring Sexual Lives and Respectful Relationships. *Journal of Gay & Lesbian Social Services* 32: 354–376. https://doi.org/10.1080/10538720.2020.1752875.

McCarthy, Michelle. 2014. Women with Intellectual Disability: Their Sexual Lives in the 21st Century. *Journal of Intellectual & Developmental Disability* 39: 124–131.

Milner, Paul, Brigit Mirfin-Veitch, Kelly Tikao, and Patsie Frawley. 2019. *"Mean As!" The Story of Creating an Online Library About Relationships and Sexuality Told and Read by Whaikaha Māori and Men and Women with a Learning Disability*. Dunedin, New Zealand: Donald Beasley Institute. https://www.donaldbeasley.org.nz/assets/projects/Mean-As/Mean-As-Academic-Report.pdf. Accessed on 18 September 2024.

Mirfin-Veitch, Brigit, Kelly Tikao, Umi Asaka, Eden Tuisaula, Hilary Stace, Robbie F. Watene, and Frawley Patsie. 2022. *Tell Me About You: A Life Story Approach to Understanding Disabled People's Experiences in Care (1950–1999)*. Dunedin, New Zealand: Donald Beasley Institute.

Office of National Statistics. 2019. *Disability and Crime, UK: 2019*. London: Office of National Statistics. https://www.ons.gov.uk/peoplepopulationandcommunity/healthandsocialcare/disability/bulletins/disabilityandcrimeuk/2019. Accessed on 18 September 2024.

O'Mahony, Charles. 2023. Implementation of Article 12 of the UN Convention on the Rights of Persons with Disabilities in England and Wales and in Northern Ireland. In *Models of Implementation of Article 12 of the Convention on the Rights of Persons with Disabilities – (CRPD)*, ed. M. Domanski and B. Lackoronski, 563–586. London: Routledge.

O'Mahony, Charles, and Aisling de Paor. 2023. Implementation of Article 12 of the UN Convention on the Rights of Persons with Disabilities in Ireland. In *Models of Implementation of Article 12 of the Convention on the Rights of Persons with Disabilities (CRPD)*, ed. M. Domanski and B. Lackoronski, 297–333. London: Routledge.

O'Shea, Amie, and Patsie Frawley. 2020. Gender, Sexuality and Relationships for Young Australian Women with Intellectual Disability. *Disability & Society* 35: 654–675. https://doi.org/10.1080/09687599.2019.1647148.

Pritchard-Jones, Laura. 2018. 'Adults at risk': 'Vulnerability' By Any Other Name? *The Journal of Adult Protection* 20: 47–58. https://doi.org/10.1108/JAP-07-2017-0029.

Royal Commission of Inquiry - Abuse in Care. n.d. *Royal Commission of Inquiry - Abuse in Care*. https://www.abuseincare.org.nz/our-progress/library/v/63/statement-of-dr-brigit-mirfin-veitch. Accessed on 18 September 2024.

Scotcher, Katie. 2019. Disabled People's Basic Needs Not Met, Abuse in Care Inquiry Told. RNZ. 1 November. https://www.rnz.co.nz/news/national/402291/disabled-people-s-basic-needs-not-met-abuse-in-care-inquiry-told. Accessed on 18 September 2024.

SL&RR. n.d. *Sexual Lives & Respectful Relationships: Rights and Respect in Sexuality and Relationships*. https://web.archive.org/web/20220307020728/, https://www.slrr.com.au/. Accessed on 18 September 2024.

Sobsey, Dick. 2004. Sexual Abuse of Individuals with Intellectual Disability. In *Practice Issues in Sexuality and Learning Disability*, ed. A. Craft, 91–112. London: Routledge.

Stienstra, Deborah. 2023. (Th)reading Rights and Justice: Women and Girls with Disabilities. *Global Society* 37: 315–462.

The Equality Institute & The Accelerator for GBV Prevention. 2023. *What Counts? The State of Funding for the Prevention of Gender-based Violence Against Women and Girls*. The Equality Institute.

The Equality Institute and UN Women. 2023. *Together for Prevention: Handbook on Multisectoral National Action Plans*. New York: UN Women.

United Nations. 2006. Convention on the Rights of Persons With Disabilities. New York: United Nations. https://www.ohchr.org/en/instruments-mechanisms/instruments/convention-rights-persons-disabilities. Accessed on 18 September 2024.

World Health Organisation. n.d. *World Health Organisation - Violence Prevention Alliance*. https://www.who.int/groups/violence-prevention-alliance/approach#:~:text=The%20ecological%20framework,-The%20ecological%20framework&text=This%20framework%20views%20interpersonal%20violence,the%20community%2C%20and%20the%20societal. Accessed on 18 September 2024.

World Health Organisation. n.d. *World Health Organisation- Violence Prevention Approach*. https://www.who.int/violenceprevention/approach/ecology/en/. Accessed on 18 September 2024.

# Medical Knowledge in Forensic Settings

# Racialisation in the Court and Clinic: Controlling Images, Black Motherhood and Sexual Assault Forensic Intervention

*Sameena Mulla and Heather R. Hlavka*

## 1 Introduction: Race and Sexual Assault Intervention

When prosecuting sexual assault, the court of law operates in many registers of justice. In the US and other jurisdictions, the practice of law is not simply concerned with formally settling questions of responsibility or guilt in response to allegations of sexual harm, but also reproduces broader cultural narratives which give order to race, gender, class, and sexuality. In the Milwaukee County Circuit Courts, where we conducted

---

Authors are listed in reverse alphabetical order and are equal contributors to this work.

---

S. Mulla (✉)
Emory University, Atlanta, USA
e-mail: sameena.mulla@emory.edu

H. R. Hlavka
Marquette University, Milwaukee, USA
e-mail: heather.hlavka@marquette.edu



R. E. Keyse et al. (eds.), *Sexual Violence in Medicine and Psychiatry*, Genders and Sexualities in History,
https://doi.org/10.1007/978-3-032-10800-5_6

field research from 2013 to 2016, we often recalled Ruha Benjamin's observation that adjudication was a carceral technology that served to 'fix in place' trial participants (Benjamin 2016). In this chapter, we consider the ways in which the inclusion of expert knowledges by forensic nurses, medical personnel, and attorneys were among the carceral technologies that surveilled Blackness. In the proceedings we observed, it was primarily the victim-witness around whom knowledge was produced, and whose experiences were the central focus of the trial. We read the carceral technologies through which victim-witness experience was interpreted as comprising the apparatus of racialising surveillance, and focus on how Black women and girls were subjected to these technologies and the deep histories that attended them. We therefore argue that sexual assault adjudication and its reliance on and reification of forensic technique served to police racial boundaries. Focusing on the Milwaukee County Court System in Milwaukee, Wisconsin, USA, we show how these forces operated within US jurisprudence and suggest that the role of forensic science as a carceral technology operates in many sexual assault intervention settings and across distinctive racial and (post)-colonial regimes with their own unique histories. In particular, racial surveillance is rooted in both carceral and clinical regimes.

In *Dark Matters,* Simone Browne defined racialising surveillance as 'a technology of social control where surveillance practices, policies, and performances concern the production of norms pertaining to race and a "power to define what is in or out of place"' (Browne 2015, 16). These modes of surveillance encompassed technologies that 'reify boundaries, borders, and bodies along racial lines', and resulted in 'discriminatory treatment of those who are negatively racialised' (Ibid). We read Browne's account as an operation of 'jurisgenerativity', what Robert Cover explained was 'the work of courts, which commonly inhibit—but occasionally foster—the processes of creating legal meaning' (Cover 1983, 26). Jurisgenerativity is often defined as generating legal meaning within legal institutions, but law itself is an authoritative realm of knowledge production and thus can generate meaning that transcends the courts. The legal meanings we explore in this chapter are generated at the intersections of witness testimony and forensic discourse. We argue that in the US trial, forensic science increases the capacity of jurisgenerativity, contributing racialising logics and empowering its own racial ordering. Forensic narratives do not solely focus on the defendant. Rather, victim-witnesses are entangled in the formal rules of the court and the production of expert testimony. Collectively, these technologies cast Black women and girls as pathological maternal figures, or hypersexualised and manipulative, while reinscribing white forms of maternity and sexuality as normative. These characterisations are rooted in what Patricia Hill Collins termed, 'controlling images' (1990, 67).

In the first section of this chapter, we discuss the framework of controlling images, their historical context, and how we saw them relating to US legal regimes that circulated within the courtroom during sexual assault trials. We then turn to how clinical practices upon which sexual assault adjudication focused were themselves fraught with a racial politics inherited from clinical regimes. Additionally, the role of enslaved Black women as experimental subjects and nurses in gynaecology's history shaped a conscripted range of agency for the contemporary gynaecological patient. In the third section, we turn to how this patient could be subjected to the forensic interpretation of their body and experience when entering the courts. While the advent of sexual assault reforms that gave rise to forensic nursing professionalisation may have improved the quality of care for some patients, it did not address the broader structural components of anti-Black racism. In the final section, we work through the way powerful controlling images of Black motherhood surfaced within the course of the trial. The pathologisation of Black motherhood was sustained by both legal and clinical tropes that intersect in the courts. In the conclusion, we discuss how the courts relied on both legal and clinical practices that were ingrained with the racialising regimes of colonialism and chattel slavery. We end with the caution that a path to sexual assault intervention as liberatory practice must disrupt the court's deep history of racial surveillance. To recognise this racial surveillance, we must cultivate a scepticism that regards both clinical and legal practices as perpetuating harm.

## 2 Controlling Images and the Law

In the opening of her well-known chapter on controlling images in *Black Feminist Thought*, Patricia Hill Collins began with an epigraph from literary scholar Trudier Harris.

Harris wrote,

> Called Matriarch, Emasculator and Hot Momma. Sometimes Sister, Pretty Baby, Auntie, Mammy and Girl. Called Unwed Mother, Welfare Recipient and Inner City Consumer. The Black American Woman has had to admit

> that while nobody knew the troubles she saw, everybody, his brother and his dog, felt qualified to explain her, even to herself. (Harris 1982, 4, as cited in Collins 1990, 67)

Where Harris introduced this commentary in the realm of representing Black domestic workers in American literature, Collins cast these explanations of Black womanhood from the literary into the sociological. She termed these iconic stereotypes 'controlling images', explaining them as part of a 'generalised ideology of domination', whose very purpose was to serve as an 'instrument of power' (Collins 1990, 68). After detailing the four most common archetypes circulating as controlling images, Collins further identified institutional sites as 'essential for transmitting ideologies objectifying Black woman as the Other' (Collins 1990, 85). Although Collins named the role of institutions, particularly schools, the media, corporations and government agencies, as central in the transmission of controlling images, she did not write *Black Feminist Thought* as the place to undertake an institutional analysis. Rather, one purpose of the work comprised a set of tools to practise Black feminist thought. Following her invitation, we ask what possibilities unfold if we consider the courts as an institution mobilising controlling images, where forensic experts, police, and lawyers trade in explaining Black women's sexuality to settle the question of an allegation of sexual assault? When are Collins's controlling images to be found in the court of law itself? How do these images contribute to the jurisgeneration of anti-Blackness?

Having their origins in different moments of US history, Collin's work highlighted four controlling images including the Mammy, Matriarch, Welfare Mother, and Jezebel. Each controlling image fixed Black women in specific frameworks with regards to maternity and sexuality. Collins also carefully pointed out that while the images often worked simultaneously, they also created untenable positions for Black women to occupy. For example, the Mammy archetype was drawn from the period in which Black women were forced to labour as enslaved domestic workers and invest their maternal energies into the children of slave owners rather than their own children. The Mammy was therefore a desexualised figure, which stood in stark contrast with the Matriarch, Welfare Mother and Jezebel, who were often ascribed with hypersexuality (Collins 1990, 71). Where the Mammy was not allowed to mother her own children, the Matriarch was seen as a single head of household who overpowered and expelled Black men, a cultural orientation resulting from the tearing apart of Black families as a result of chattel slavery. Because slavery divided enslaved people from their children and partners, the theory of the controlling image of the Mammy and Matriarch asserted that Black women developed a steely self-reliance in the absence of their menfolk. In the post-Emancipation period, Black women were further pathologised through the claim they were unable to share the head of household role with men, the earlier matriarch role having calcified into stereotypes about the way Black women mothered and ran households.

Following World War II, the Welfare Mother emerged as a controlling image of a Black woman who participated in a maternity alleged to instrumentalise her children as conduits to the largess of state benefits (Collins 1990, 76). Though the historical periods in which these controlling images were born were long past, Collins noted their persistence even as they had no empirical foundation. Thinking through the cultural narratives about Black women that percolate within the space and practices of US sexual assault adjudication, it bears mentioning Patricia Williams's observation that,

> Blacks and women are the objects of a constitutional omission which has been incorporated into a theory of neutrality. It is thus that omission is really a form of expression, as oxymoronic as that sounds: racial omission is a literal part of original intention; it is the fixed, reiterated prophecy of the Founding Fathers. (Williams 1989, 2142-2143).

In short, the law itself was authored with the intent of excluding Black women. Historically, there were no legal sanctions for sexual violence against Black women (Donovan and Williams 2002; Pokorak 2006). For example, many southern US state laws of the nineteenth century were race-specific, many of which only legally recognised white women as subject to rape (Sommerville 2004; Thompson 2021). When Black women found themselves subject to legal protections, they were juxtaposed against the images of white women as virginal and virtuous. This was always necessarily a project of retrofitting Black women into legal mores which were not crafted with the intent of affording them legal rights, particularly in relationship to rape (Roberts 1997, 31). The period of chattel slavery was, of course, defined by the brutal control over Black women's sexuality and reproductive capacity that essentialised them as 'unrapeable' in a legal sense (Pokorak 2006). As Crenshaw states, 'Their femaleness made them sexually vulnerable to racist domination, while their Blackness effectively denied them any protection' (1989, 159).

We now understand that this landscape of sexual terror persisted beyond emancipation, and Black communities were deeply aware that local authorities would do little to protect them from sexual violence. Rather than wait for the law to protect them, Black civic associations often mobilised to investigate such crimes themselves, perhaps best exemplified in the National Association for the Advancement of Colored People's deployment of Rosa Parks to investigate the kidnapping and rape of Recy Taylor in 1944 (McGuire 2017). Following the civil rights movements of the 1960s, Black Americans were encouraged to rely more heavily on legal and criminal justice institutions, as though the racial disparities of the past might dramatically cease to exist. Writing about Black women's experiences of sexual violence in the Midwest, scholar Darlene Clark Hine traced how the attendant stakes of formally disclosing rape led to a culture of reticence (Hine 1989, 914). Coming forward was simply too risky, exposing rape victims to the state, threatening livelihoods, and opening communities to carceral scrutiny.

In one of the two articles in which legal scholar Kimberlé Crenshaw named and described intersectionality, she specifically explored how race and gender worked together to inflect women of color's experiences of rape in US law (Crenshaw 1991, 1245). By tracing the discursive life of the controlling image into the forensic setting, this chapter takes up Crenshaw's call to examine the particular stakes of Black women navigating criminal justice institutions. Legal adjudication of sexual assault in the U.S., as well as many other jurisdictions outside of the U.S., routinely includes forensic expertise (Hlavka and Mulla 2020). This forensic expertise manifests as testimony from forensic nurses, forensic scientists, and police. It is also woven into the arguments of attorneys and the rhetoric of judges. Anthropologist Brendane Tynes has noted that sexual assault intervention as a process linked to the courts, is deeply invested in controlling images (Tynes 2022). In the next sections, we show how fragments of controlling images that assign Black women to a subordinate status emerged within the rhetoric and testimony of forensic nurses. Here, we return to Harris's complaint that Black women and girls found themselves being explained. Despite Black women and girls own testimony provided as victim-witnesses at trial, forensic expertise often stood in to narrate explanations of Black women's troubles.

## 3 Sexual Assault, Evidence Collection, and Gynaecology's History

While contemporary sexual assault statutes in the US lay claim to race neutrality, the history of law can itself be read as a project of racial domination. For example, an 1859 Mississippi Supreme Court ruling, *George v. State*, determined that a Black man could only commit rape against a white woman (Estrich 1987). While such laws have been superseded over time, the law continues to play a role in criminalising sexual assault along racial lines. These racial lines are monitored not only through statutory language and case law, but in contemporary contexts through the law's dependence on forensic expertise. One of the primary explanatory modalities of sexual assault adjudication is through forensic intervention. In her discussion of carceral imaginaries, Ruha Benjamin explained that carceral technologies are

> not only applicable to those processes that are directly tied to prisons and police; rather, I propose an expansive understanding of containment that trains scholarly attention to the underside of technoscientific development— who and what are fixed in place— classified, corralled, and/or coerced, to enable innovation? In the postracial era, subjugation is hardly ever the explicit objective of science and technology; instead, noble aims such as 'health' and 'safety' serve as a kind of moral prophylaxis for newfangled forms of classification and control (Benjamin 2016, 150).

Focusing on the use of spirometry in measuring lung capacity, Benjamin described how the health care workers who rely on the technology are often unaware of how it 'corrects' for race. With or without their knowledge, they reproduced a racist practice that normalises lower lung capacities for Black and brown patients. The consequences of these practices were primarily borne by patients of colour, who had to reach a higher threshold of respiratory distress to warrant intervention as compared to white patients.

Forensic examination is the primary technology of evidence in sexual assault adjudication and introduces a technoscientific deployment of classification that knits together the clinic and the court. Thinking with Benjamin's terms, we can characterise sexual assault medico-legal examination as a clinical regime of coercion and corralling (Doe 2012; Mulla 2014). Andrea Quinlan characterised the exam as far from 'a neutral object' as it recruits victim-survivors into a set of practices with a long and complex history (Quinlan 2017, 12). One of the most sobering strands to unravel lies in the origins of forensic intervention: in its heavy reliance on pelvic examination, sexual assault examination draws on gynaecology. The techniques of gynaecology have been critically interrogated by scholars who recognise that the experimental context of American chattel slavery gave rise to the speculum, the development of the lithotomy position, and many gynaecological surgical techniques (Cooper Owens 2017; Dudley 2012; Kapsalis 1997). In noting the expectations that the ideal gynaecology patient was silent, submissive, and unobtrusive, while unable to see the examination of her pelvis which was covered by a draped sheet at the waist, sociologists Henslin and Biggs did not name the origins of US gynaecological practice as it is rooted in the history of slavery (1971). 'The ghost of these histories seemed to assert itself in the submission and acquiescence that forensic nurses often expected from people undergoing pelvic examinations' (Mulla 2023, 156), and it is instructive to think about the submission that has been characteristically expected of the patient undergoing pelvic examination. Is the gynaecological patient's submission an artefact of the enslaved status of women such as Anarcha, Betsy and Lucy, and about nine other women whose names are lost to us, who served as the unconsenting subjects of J. Marion Sims's obstetric experiments (Cooper Owens 2017; Dudley 2012)?

Historian Deirdre Cooper Owens also documents the labors of Anarcha, Betsy, Lucy and their companions recovering from Sims's experimental procedures, but this part of gynaecological history is often erased in clinical settings, including in the sexual assault forensic examination. The submission to gynaecologic intervention must also be contextualised within the framework of labour, value, and 'repair'. That is, Sims negotiated access to his experimental subjects because slave owners were concerned about

> returning enslaved women to their full capacity to labor for slave owners. These labors were both as producers and as household workers, as well as reproductive laborers whose reproductive capacity could be exploited and alienated (Mulla 2023, 156).

The phantoms of gynaecology's history haunt contemporary notions of patient compliance and cooperation. Conforming to the ideal of being a good patient is often incorporated into what nurses perceive as a 'good victim' (Mulla 2014).

In the 1970s, forensic nursing emerged as a specialisation in the US building on anti-rape movements. Crenshaw, however, noted that 'reforms of rape law and judicial procedures that are premised on narrow conceptions of gender subordination may not address the devaluation of Black women' (1991, 1270). Sexual Assault Nurse Examiner (SANE) programs began the work of professionalising forensic nurses by training them in collecting forensic evidence and providing clinical and emotional care for rape victims (Ledray 1999; Campbell 2006). At the time of writing this chapter, forensic nursing requires intense training and staffing, and as such, SANE programs are overwhelmingly located at urban hospitals in the US, where such staffing needs can be supported. Forensic nursing emerges at the confluence of nursing practice and criminal justice adjudication, and nurses who conduct examinations of patients may testify in court to their documented clinical and forensic interactions and findings. Recall of course, that forensic nurses typically testified in a very small number of sexual assault cases and were more likely to testify to the absence rather than the presence of forensic evidence (Hlavka and Mulla 2021). The public imaginary of SANE programs and forensic evidence often failed to account for how technoscience is recruited into the liberal US project of the condemnation of Blackness through its deployment of institutional expertise, efficiency, and 'race neutral' evaluations (Muhammad 2010). Despite its claims of race neutrality, Black women experienced a sense of dehumanisation in their experiences of sexual assault forensic intervention (Ruiz et al. 2023).

Rose Corrigan's research on SANE programs provides an important critique, detailing how the development of these programs have created 'new' obstacles for rape survivors such as police obstruction, disproportionate scrutiny of victim credibility, and decreased access to medical care (Corrigan 2013a, b). Terming the SANE exam as a 'trial by ordeal'—a 'test' of one's credibility—Corrigan expertly described how rape complainants can be judged by their compliance and cooperation to undergo the forensic exam and thus enter into a coerced relationship with the criminal justice system. Therefore, one person's 'commitment' to the justice system may cast suspicion on those rape victims who decided not to participate in medical or forensic interventions. This participation may well be rooted in the disparate treatment Black women experience at the hands of the court, and even in the clinic. It is useful to recall Crenshaw's concern that the very systems that Black women rely upon to navigate sexual violence include racist institutions whose racism is not suspended simply because Black women and other women of color occupy the subject position of 'victim' (Crenshaw 1991). Recent studies have demonstrated that these inequalities continue to shape the way Black women balance the risks of medical and policing interventions when they are sexually assaulted (Kelley 2023).

While SANE programs have improved access to care for some survivors, research on Black women's experiences of post-assault interventions, including forensic examination, medical treatment, access to emergency conception, prophylaxis for infections, legal advocacy, and follow up care are rarely contextualised. Sociohistorical contexts may explain why some researchers have found that Black women have negative experiences with medical and advocacy professionals during sexual assault interventions (Maier 2008; Washington 2001). Corrigan reminds us that

> Forensic evidence does not provide a meaningful check on individual or systemic biases [...] lessons from history should remind scholars to be skeptical about whether such technologies really are a step forward in some teleological progress toward truth and certainty in the criminal justice process. Ostensibly scientific (and therefore neutral, objective, and fair) tools can mask individual and cultural interests in how such tools constitute evidence and therefore procure legal outcomes. (2013a, 944-45)

While rape victims are often burdened by the circulation of rape myths and negative stereotypes during interactions with SANE nurses and criminal justice personnel, Roxanne Donovan and Michelle Williams have found that Black women are additionally burdened by controlling images characterising them as 'promiscuous', which Donovan and Williams describe as a 'double dose of rape myths' (2002, 98). Additionally, Black women face the challenges of denial of medical services and shelter based on provider's perceptions of their strength and resilience (Bent-Goodley 2004; Donnelly et al. 1999). Black women's reports of sexual violence are often met with scepticism and are not deemed worthy of a response from law enforcement (Crenshaw 1991; Donnelly et al. 1999; Potter 2010). Instead, victims may experience discrimination and harsh interrogations by hospital staff, and uneven services from care providers (Campbell and Raja 2005). For example, Campbell and colleagues found that Black women (40%) were provided with less information about HIV from forensic nurses than were white women (60%) (Campbell et al. 2008). In this example, uneven care was aligned with differential interpretations of the sexual assault complainant as a knowledge-worthy subject.

## 4 Forensic Interpretation of Black Women's Bodies

Injury detection and underreporting were another area that disproportionately impacts Black women navigating forensic intervention. Studies on anogenital injury prevalence and frequency found significant effects between different races, ethnicities, and skin colour variances (Baker et al. 2010; Cartwright 1987; Sommers et al. 2008). In short, race and skin colour were significantly associated with the frequency of injuries documented in medical records and in forensic nurse examinations. Research found differences in injury based on race, with white women documented as more likely to sustain injury than Black women including occurrence and frequency in the external genitalia such as the thighs, labia majora, posterior fourchette, and fossa navicularis (Baker et al. 2010; Sommers et al. 2008). Therefore, women with 'dark skin will not be as likely as those with light skin to have their injuries identified, documented, and treated' (Sommers et al. 2008). And Baker and colleagues explicitly linked these findings to court, stating that forensic nurses needed to explain on the stand that injuries in women of colour were detected less frequently than with white women:

> When injuries are considered as forensic evidence, it is important that the associations among injuries, race, and color are acknowledged...until the science behind the forensic examination is advanced, it is crucial that other parts of the testimony, including the victims statement about the rape, are considered equally important, if not more important, than the injuries documented. (2010, 150)

During our fieldwork, we did not observe any forensic nurses testifying to the scientific literature documenting variances in forensic examination injury detection based on racial, ethnic, or skin colour variations, nor was it mentioned by forensic nurses in the 22 interviews conducted during our study (Hlavka and Mulla 2021). Attorneys largely called on forensic nurses to testify as fact witnesses, and that testimony tended to provide jurors with lessons on genital anatomy, while reading and reviewing forensic examination reports.

Presenting themselves as objective and institutional, forensic nurses offered 'race-neutral' evaluations centred around heteronormative constructions of female anatomy and reproductive norms. Race-neutrality, however, invited the jury and court personnel to project their own racial knowledge and prejudice onto the victim-witness. During court, they often described vaginas as 'stretchy'; 'lubricated'; 'strong'; 'self-cleaning'; 'quick to heal'; and 'made to have sexual intercourse'. The vagina was described as normal/healthy or abnormal/unhealthy. Abnormality was linked to illness, nutrition, poverty, or to child-like ignorance. Nurses' testimony was interpellated into the trial to produce symbolic representations of 'normal' heteronormative, white bodies to which Black bodies were to be compared. Black women and girls' injuries, or lack of injuries, were explained and interpreted by attorneys as indicative of hygienic maladaptation, feminised bodily functions (e.g. miscarriages, menstruation), multiple sex partners, evidence of consensual sex, or evidence that, despite testimony to the contrary, the assault did not take place at all. Thus, we argue, 'the authority of witness as embodied by forensic nurses rendering Black girls' suffering bodies legible to the court suggests the racial regimes of producing knowledge of sexual violence' (Hlavka and Mulla 2021, 149).

In our work on children's credibility in court, we noted how defence attorneys alleged that some of the witnesses practised poor hygiene, and this resulted in genital injuries. This argument acted as racialising tropes to position a young Black girl's body as dirty and poor in sharp contrast with a clean middle-class white body (Powell et al. 2017). Both our fieldnotes and official trial transcripts are replete with questions from attorneys calling for explanations of women's bodies—be it their hygiene rituals, menstrual cycles, miscarriages, or sexual activity and histories. For example, in Jessica's[1] case—a young, seven-year-old Black girl, a nurse documented redness to her hymen. While the prosecution argued that the redness was consistent with sexual assault, defense argued it could have been 'caused by poor hygiene', 'infection' or 'wiping too much' with 'toilet paper that is too rough' (467). The interpretation of poor hygiene and self-harm invokes a controlling image of a poor, ignorant, but precocious child, which conflicts with the controlling image of the strong and sturdy Black woman. The discrepancies between controlling images

[1] This, and all names in cases cited from our field project, are pseudonyms and all identifying characteristics have been removed.

that are simultaneously deployed within particular institutional sites, like courts, are part of the practice of racial ordering.

Following the forensic nurse's testimony and commentary of the victim-witness's body, other courtroom actors were then able to participate in these interpretive practices even without the mantle of forensic expertise. In the case of a 27-year-old Black woman, L'umoya, the defence attorney questioned everything about L'umoya's body—from her miscarriage to her body size ('…she weighs 206 pounds, so she's not a small person') to her 'tight red jeans, [her] blue and white hair extensions'' and 'pink thong underwear' and the very neighbourhood in which she lived ('..the area of Lisbon Avenue…she knows that's a prostitution area') (Hlavka and Mulla 2021, 254). Public discourses about Black women's sexual availability and relationship to reproduction circulated broadly within lay and medical imaginaries. Here, the court became the site of invoking the controlling image of the Jezebel. Additionally, the court oriented towards Black women and girls as inscrutable and mysterious, requiring the (most often white) nurse's translational techniques and testimony to make injuries legible by reminding juries about principles of health and human capacities in general terms.

In L'umoya's case, she had flagged down a passing police car after fleeing from her abductors, later going to the hospital for a SANE examination. The forensic nurse testified at trial that L'umoya complained of great pain to her arms, neck, and mouth, 'a level eight on a 10-point scale'. The nurse said, 'when I touched her, she cringed or moved away from the touch'. Still, no visible injuries were documented on the exterior of her body. The nurse had not seen any bruising or swelling. These injuries, however, were more likely to show up hours to days after an assault. The nurse did, however, document injury to L'umoya's perihymenal tissue and when asked by the prosecutor what might have caused the injury, the SANE nurse responded, 'the vagina does not just tear on its own. That tissue is strong. If someone has an infection and things like that, that could make your skin more prone to tear on its own'. The nurse saw herself as giving a balanced response, explaining that physical injury was a likely cause to the tear, but that infection could also be a factor. On cross-examination, the defence attorney asked the nurse more questions about these injuries:

| | |
|---|---|
| Defence counsel | The tear we're talking about, you measured it, right? |
| SANE nurse | Yes. |
| Defence | How big was it? |
| SANE | Less than a millimetre. |
| Defence | And you said it could be caused by penis to vagina intercourse, correct? |
| SANE | Yes. |
| Defence | Normally, though, that doesn't cause an injury, though, penis to vagina intercourse? |
| SANE | Yes. |
| Defence | People have sex all the time, they don't get injuries from it? |
| SANE | Correct. |
| Defence | Now, what else could cause a less than one millimetre tear like this in that area? |
| SANE | I can't think of anything off the top of my head. I'm sorry. |
| Defence | Does hygiene have anything to do with what might happen like this? |
| SANE | If there was infection to the tissue, you could have a tear. |
| Defence | Right. Does her menstrual cycle have an effect or wearing tampons or other feminine products that might dehydrate the area? |
| SANE | The area where the injury was is more sterile, so that's less likely, but I couldn't say a hundred percent what caused that injury. |
| Defence | Right, and it was near that posterior fourchette area you talked about? |
| SANE | Yes. |
| Defence | But that area itself has no injury, correct? |
| SANE | Correct. |
| Defence | And this you said had no drainage from it? |
| SANE | Correct. |
| Defence | No bleeding or anything like that? |
| SANE | Correct. |

Later during cross-examination, the defence attorney again asked the SANE nurse to clarify that she '... can't tell exactly when that tear appeared, correct?' asking more questions about the possibility of previous infection:

| | |
|---|---|
| Defence | Just real quick. I know you said you didn't see any signs of infection in the vaginal area, correct? |
| SANE | Correct. |
| Defence | But you didn't see any symptoms of infections right? |
| SANE | I did not see any symptoms of infection, correct. |
| Defence | To actually know if there is an infection or not, you have to do blood work, correct? |
| SANE | Or genital tests, yes, you would have to do some sort of testing for infection. |

Once more, the defence had attempted to cast doubt on the origin of L'umoya's injuries. His questions minimised the injuries, and insisted on the uncertainty of rape as the cause of injury. There could be no conclusive observations here. Raising the spectre of infection cast L'umoya as potentially diseased, even pathologically unclean. While the nurse herself was careful to explain that infection had also not been detected, the defence attorney succeeded in having the nurse spend a disproportionate amount of time discussing these possibilities. Given the allegations that the defence attorney raised suggesting that L'umoya was a sex worker, the insinuation he aimed for may well have been to suggest she had sexually transmitted infections, thus linking forensics with the controlling image of the Jezebel. These insinuations seemed toothless to us as we observed the trial, but in later months when we reviewed the transcript, we realised that the sceptical faces of the jurors were erased from the transcript and what persisted instead was a disjointed and decontextualised account of the defence's questions; a transcript now fixed into legal record. It is also important to note that all along, L'umoya had been clear to communicate with the nurse about her injuries. She never cited illness as a possibility, while she had indicated that she was in pain because she had been sexually assaulted. In the court, however, the nurse and the attorneys asserted their own interpretations of L'umoya's pain and injury.

## 5 What Kind of Mother: Black Motherhood and Sexual Violence

Like many of the women in the courts, L'umoya was a mother, and motherhood was another area open to a great deal of interpretation during adjudication. Motherhood is also central to the discourses of controlling images. The sexual and moral degradation of Black mothers during sexual assault trials produced a racial hierarchy that degraded Black women, negatively comparing them to forms of motherhood embedded in white heteronormativity. In the trials we observed, both defence counsel and the prosecution capitalised on controlling images such as the promiscuous sex worker, 'welfare mother', 'baby mama', or 'Jezebel' (Collins 2000; see Powell et al. 2017). These controlling images and racialising scripts were deployed in varying ways, dependent upon the age and role of the victim-witness. For example, Black mothers were regularly portrayed as vindictive, 'poisonous', and manipulative. Counsel often argued that mothers had pressured their daughters to lie and report they were abused by their (step)fathers. In other cases, Black mothers were exploited to enhance defence attorney's arguments for their client's innocence. During our fieldwork we were told of 'unsupportive' Black mothers who did not believe their child/ren's testimony. In some cases, the allegations had resulted in children being removed to foster care homes, breaking up families and separating siblings. Prosecutors often signalled disapproval or disgust with unfit mothers, while defence attorneys easily took advantage in closing arguments, such as in one trial where the attorney stated:

> Ladies and gentlemen, if her own mother doesn't believe her, why should you? Her own mother who she lives with doesn't believe her. I have got two daughters. If they came to me and said somebody sexually assaulted 'em, I would believe 'em. Doesn't mean it is true, but I would believe them. Her own mother doesn't believe her.

Black mothers as victim-witnesses, as in the cases of Mary, Tamee, and L'umoya described below, were commonly characterised as representing deviant womanhood which challenged white, hegemonic femininity (Richie 2012; Powell et al. 2017). Indeed, prosecutors often repeated the common refrain that 'mom's boyfriend' was the major threat against children. This refrain demonstrated the precariousness of mothering. Court counsel engaged these intersecting narratives in several powerful ways. Invoking various controlling images, they called into question Black mothers' roles, decision-making, and livelihoods.

In one case, Mary's testimony of being sexually assaulted by her former partner, Jerry, revealed some complicated details of their previous relationship. Jerry was the father of her six-year-old child, and she was a home health care worker and payee for Jerry's Social Security payments. Their relationship had been over for quite some time prior to the assault, and Mary was the primary caregiver to their child. She also was tasked with regularly visiting Jerry to help him with his care. The defence attorney described Mary as a 'single mother' in low-income employment. Because of this precarity, the attorney argued that Mary had offered sex to Jerry in exchange for money—like the many transactional sex defences we witnessed during our field observations in cases involving Black victims and defendants (Hlavka and Mulla 2021). Without evidence to support his claim, defence counsel further suggested that Mary was jealous of Jerry's interest in another woman, interweaving controlling images of the Matriarch, Welfare Mother, and Jezebel with regards to maternity and sexuality (Collins 1990).

In another case that we have written about at length, the maternal qualities of Tamee North came under aspersion (Hlavka and Mulla 2018, 2021). Tamee alleged that her ex-boyfriend, Kelvin Lee, with whom she shared children, had threatened her with sexual assault at gunpoint. During the trial, we listened to the prosecutor read dozens of text message exchanges in which Kelvin degraded and insulted Tamee (Hlavka and Mulla 2018). Defence counsel portrayed Kelvin as a doting father caught in the vindictiveness of his ex-girlfriend's lies. Tamee, on the other hand, was characterised as promiscuous and disreputable. Tamee and Kelvin shared custody, and she supported herself and her children as a dancer and performer at an adult venue. Tamee's 'scandalous' profession was repeatedly called into question, used to characterise her as a Jezebel, and bad mother. In particular, the court vilified Tamee's dancing profession rather than classifying it as a creative or resourceful way to secure her own living and that of her children. Despite clear testimony and corroborating evidence to show that Kelvin had threatened sexual assault of Tamee at gunpoint, witnesses who described her as 'weeping' and 'crying' in the aftermath of the assault, and forensic photographs of Tamee with visible scratches on her chest, the jury found the defendant not guilty of the crimes.

A few weeks later, as we were entering a courtroom, the judge who had presided over the same case was hurriedly exiting. We had a brief opportunity to ask her if she had any notes or observations about State vs. Kelvin Lee, knowing that these sorts of passing conversations were often less guarded than our formal recorded interviews. The judge immediately expressed her offended sensibilities: 'What kind of mother', she opined, would act the way Tamee had acted? Why would she work as a dancer and send such obscenity-filled text messages? As the judge exited the courtroom, we could see she was exasperated, and from her perspective, her statement required no further explanation. Tamee's credibility centred on roles as co-parent and mother. The defence attorney consistently called her morality into question, casting her as angry, sexually promiscuous, and unfeminine (Hlavka and Mulla 2018). Tamee did not conform to the rules of white, heteronormative respectability and was thus cast accordingly whereby her words and text messages were weaponised against her and she was deemed 'unrapeable'. In this brief exchange with the judge, it was clear she had framed Tamee's credibility as related to her 'bad' mothering, despite the lack of evidence about Tamee's mothering presented at trial. And there were no similar recriminations for Kelvin and his fathering in the judge's quick criticism. Rather, the judge's criticism mirrored the defendant's language on the stand and in the text messages presented to the court in troubling, superficial ways. Perhaps we had expected some discussion of how hard such allegations were to prove in these types of cases, or the interesting way in which text messages had been used during the trial? Instead, we were left to wonder 'what kind of mother' Tamee was in the eyes of the judge.

Turning back to L'umoya's case, the fact of her motherhood was largely minimised. As noted in the previous section, L'umoya's gruelling testimony described the night the defendant, a stranger to her, and one of his accomplices abducted her off the street and sexually assaulted her. Again, the defence suggested this was no kidnapping, but simply an instance of transactional sex. Why else would L'umoya be walking at night in 'that area' of Milwaukee? Though most of these details were mentioned outside of the jurors' hearing, we knew from speaking with the prosecutor and attending earlier pre-trial hearings that L'umoya had an agonising year post-assault. During her testimony, the prosecutor asked what she was wearing that night. Replying that she was dressed in 'a green hoodie I wore all the time', details of her fixation with the hooded jacket were not addressed at trial but became clearer during the sentencing hearing. During the sentencing of the defendant, the prosecutor described L'umoya as in a profound state of depression following the assault. Noting for the court record that she was unable to physically leave her house to attend the hearing and deliver a victim impact statement, the prosecutor revealed that during the trial, a Milwaukee police officer and a social worker had to accompany L'umoya to court given her paralysing fear. The prosecutor then further explained the extent of her suffering in relation to her mothering:

She still is unable to leave her house. She was wearing a hoodie all around her house all the time, and her son thought that the hoodie was making her so sad because he observed her to be so sad and distraught after this incident that her son threw the hoodie away because in his young mind the hoodie was causing her to be so sad that if he threw it away, it would make her feel better. That's how profound this crime has affected [her]. She can't look people in the eye, she can't leave her house. She lost her job. She's in total isolation.... Her fear of being out in public has affected how she is parenting her son. She doesn't want him to leave either, which is having a great effect on him. The whole family has noticed the deep and profound sadness.

The sentencing judge then described L'umoya as 'shrouded in a hoodie' and experiencing extreme trauma that 'also victimised her child'. Most of these details were not revealed during trial, and the jury only heard brief mention that L'umoya had a 12-year-old son. In addition, there was no mention of L'umoya's reproductive history or status as a mother in the testimony of other witnesses. This omission is an interesting (and consistent one) when considering the testimony of SANE nurses, who described pelvic examinations from the stand in rather generic, but heteronormative terms—rendering the vagina as 'stretchy' and 'reproductive'. While SANE nurses are often trained to describe the appearance of the cervix in relationship to pregnancy, discerning between 'parous' or 'nulliparous' status (International Association of Forensic Nursing 2013), they rarely explain these details when testifying. Nor do they offer fact evidence for whether the patient had ever been pregnant or given birth (a question routinely asked of patients during intake for the hospital examination).

Such omissions contribute both to the inscrutability of motherhood on the stand, and to the ways in which motherhood is highly interpretable within the courts. While this inscrutability is no doubt sustained by the imperative to maintain a patient's privacy, it can also contribute to the dehumanisation of the victim-witness. In this case, L'umoya had been walking from her house to her mother's house and back to pick up some medications she needed.

> Her asthma pump, her son's asthma pump, and pain pills she was taking after a recent miscarriage. Asked when she had the miscarriage, L'umoya quietly responded that '[it] happened to me my whole life'. Upon being told that she had to speak up so that the jury and the court reporter could hear her, she said: 'I lost a baby before. I just don't want to talk about that[,] please.' (Hlavka and Mulla 2021, 251)

Strands of maternal desire and thwarted pregnancy were evident when we listened to L'umoya explain why she had travelled to fetch medications in the middle of the night. Respecting L'umoya's request, the prosecutor backed away from asking further questions about her miscarriages. The defence attorney, however, capitalised on the fleeting nature of this testimony to cast doubt on why L'umoya had been out in the middle of the night if not for sex work. Curiously, Mr. Jeffers, another witness who was later called to the stand, had also left his apartment in the middle of the night to pick up prescriptions from a nearby 24-hour pharmacy. Jeffers had inadvertently interrupted the sexual assault and distracted L'umoya's attackers, which allowed her to escape. Black femininity and white masculinity were encoded differently in the courts. As a middle-aged white man, no one questioned the legitimacy of Mr. Jeffers presence in the neighbourhood. No one accused him of being a possible client or 'john', but defence suggested many times that L'umoya was a sex worker. Further, Jeffers had been shot in the arm by L'umoya's attackers, but his wound and medical visits needed no interpretation. Yet L'umoya's descriptions of her harm and pain from the sexual assault required corroboration and interpretation by the forensic nurse and a crime lab analyst. In this analysis, the conditions of L'umoya's maternity grew murkier and less discernible to the court. This dynamic, in turn, made her more vulnerable to the pathologising narrative of the defence.

## 6 Conclusion: Law, Sexual Assault and Anti-Blackness

Modern-day images of Black women and girls as promiscuous, lewd, and dishonest are rooted in US chattel slavery to justify the rape of Black women by slave owners (Collins 2004; West 2008), but what do we make of the persistence of these images and their contemporary relevance? Rather than distinguishing between sociohistorical tropes as mutually exclusive of each other, we find that courtroom practices intensify the narrative function of discrediting and pathologising Black women during sexual assault trials. This intensification relies on interlocking anti-Black cultural scripts rooted in US enslavement, which are mobilised in the expert discourses of law and forensic science. The historical lessons of gynaecology and obstetric medicine situate Black women and girls as available to the scientific and clinical gaze. While sexual assault adjudication is often analysed in relationship to its claims to seek justice, the jurisgenerativity of the courts, particularly around the charged intersection of race and gender at the heart of sexual violence, give way to the continued generation of unjust worlds. The surveillance of sexuality, tethered to the authoritative knowledge of forensic science, is one material effect of the court's investment in adjudication.

The persistence of particular narratives and their reintroduction in trial after trial as a form of truth are another aspect of sexual assault adjudication. Race and gender are wedded together as aspects of identity that are not compartmentalised into discrete categories, but are overlapping and conflicting (Cho et al. 2013). Namely, the tension between the court's insistence that it can achieve (a paternalistic) form of justice for victim-witnesses is held in tension with its commitments to anti-Blackness, which work against Black women. Hegemonic cultural narratives about Black women are perpetuated both by individuals and institutionalised in organisations, becoming embedded in structures, law, and public space (Powell et al. 2022; Ridgeway and Kricheli-Katz 2013). The institutionalisation of particular controlling images, such as the Matriarch, was exemplified in the way the courts spoke about Black mothers. When proclamations about Black maternity were offered and forensic nurses and laboratory scientists made authoritative claims, these tropes were imbued with a social force that exceeds the mere space of formal adjudication. Jurors witnessed and deliberated on the reliability of the testimony of Black women and girls, about hygiene, respectability, maternity, and the corroborative evidence of SANE nurses and material evidence.

The shaping of US practices of sexual assault adjudication with relation to a complex history of legal and clinical regimes rooted in the chattel slavery system requires particular consideration when analysing sexual harm and clinical encounters. It bears noting, however, that racialised chattel slavery is paralleled by forms of colonial law and domination in other contexts (Baxi 2014). These histories found varying regimes of legal knowledge about gender and race and sustain varying practices of surveillance.

In this chapter, we asked our readers to take seriously the way that forensic sexual assault intervention participates in the production of racist knowledge and racialising surveillance. This knowledge production process is amplified when forensic intervention becomes part of courtroom discourse. It may seem unrealistic to offer any note of hope when the anti-Blackness we describe is so insidious. Yet returning to Simone Browne, we can also consider how 'racialising surveillance created an opportunity for those constructed by such practices to resist and rebel' (Mann 2019, 77). In her description of what she terms the Captive Maternal, Joy James (2016) offered a description of the mothering practices that resist their conscription under the conditions of captivity. The particular scrutiny of Black motherhood within the courts, its elision and pathologisation, echo the mechanisms through which James described the operation of the Captive Maternal. Western theory, James wrote, was predicated on 'the diminished capacities of the captive—trauma and theft of labour and time, which legitimised the existence of Captive Maternals as inevitable, inconsequential, and invisible. Citizen and ruler benefit from reproductive labour to accrue leisure and space for theory, war, and power' (James 2016, 259).

The diminishment of the value of Black women's maternal labours in sexual assault adjudication in Milwaukee's courts may well have been of service to power. For James, Captive Maternals engage in refusals, and those refusals must be nurtured and amplified within 'autonomous zones' that 'must be defended because radical Black autonomy for freedom from empire is prohibited on plantations, in slave camps, prisons, and informal arenas of capture' (James 2023). Might the courts and the forensic examination function in this instance as informal arenas of capture and as carceral technologies? Can they be decoupled from these functions in the service to Black freedom? The abolitionist answer here would caution us that there is an ease with which controlling images fashion both legal and forensic knowledge (Tynes 2022). Sexual assault intervention under the auspices of criminal adjudication in the US is unlikely to succeed as a liberatory practice. Pressuring Black women and girls to subject themselves to forensic intervention may well be another form that the theft of labour and time takes in our carceral landscape.

**Funding** This project was funded by the National Science Foundation's Program for Law and Social Sciences (Award #1250606).

## References

Baker, Rachel, Jamison Fargo, Donna Shambley-Ebron, and Marilyn Sommers. 2010. A Source of Healthcare Disparity: Race, Skin Color, and Injuries After Rape Among Adolescents and Young Adults. *Journal of Forensic Nursing* 6: 144–150.

Baxi, Pratiksha. 2014. Sexual Violence and Its Discontents. *Annual Review of Anthropology.* 43: 139–154.

Benjamin, Ruha. 2016. Catching Our Breath: Critical Race STS and the Carceral Imagination. *Engaging Science, Technology and Society* 2: 145–156.

Bent-Goodley, Tricia. 2004. Perception of Domestic Violence: A Dialogue with African American Women. *Health and Social Work* 29: 307–316.

Browne, Simone. 2015. *Dark Matters: On the Surveillance of Blackness*. Durham: Duke University Press.

Campbell, Rebecca. 2006. Rape Survivors' Experiences with the Legal and Medical Systems: Do Rape Victim Advocates Make a Difference? *Violence against Women* 12: 30–45.

Campbell, Rebecca, and Sheela Raja. 2005. The Sexual Assault and Secondary Victimization of Female Veterans: Help-Seeking Experiences with Military and Civilian Social Systems. *Psychology of Women Quarterly* 29: 97–106.

Campbell, Jacquelyn C., M. L. Baty, R. M. Ghandour, J. K. Stockman, L. Francisco, and J. Wagman. 2008. The Intersection of Intimate Partner Violence Against Women and HIV/AIDS: A Review. *International Journal of Injury Control and Safety Promotion* 15: 221–231.

Cartwright, P. S. 1987. Factors That Correlate with Injury Sustained by Survivors of Sexual Assault. *Obstetric Gynecology* 70: 44–46.

Cho, Sumi, Kimberlé Crenshaw, and Leslie McCall. 2013. Toward a Field of Intersectionality Studies: Theory, Applications and Praxis. *Signs* 38: 785–810.

Collins, Patricia Hill. 1990. Mammies, Matriarchs and Other Controlling Images. In *Black Feminist Thought: Knowledge, Consciousness and the Politics of Empowerment*, 67–90. New York and London: Routledge.

Collins, Patricia Hill. 2000. *Black Feminist Thought: Knowledge, Consciousness, and the Politics of Empowerment*, 2nd ed. New York: Routledge.

Collins, Patricia Hill. 2004. *Black Sexual Politics: African Americans, Gender, and the New Racism*. New York: Routledge.
Corrigan, Rose. 2013a. The New Trial by Ordeal: Rape Kits, Police Practices, and the Unintended Effects of Policy Innovation. *Law and Social Inquiry* 38: 920–949.
Corrigan, Rose. 2013b. *Up Against a Wall: Rape Reform and the Failure of Success*. New York: New York University Press.
Cooper Owens, Deirdre. 2017. *Medical Bondage: Race, Gender and the Origins of American Gynecology*. Athens, GA: University of Georgia Press.
Cover, Robert. 1983. Nomos and Narrative. *Harvard Law Review* 97: 4–68.
Crenshaw, Kimberlé. 1989. Demarginalizing the Intersection of Race and Sex: A Black Feminist Critique of Antidiscrimination Doctrine, Feminist Theory and Antiracist Politics. *University of Chicago Legal Forum* 139–168.
Crenshaw, Kimberlé. 1991. Mapping the Margins: Intersectionality, Identity Politics, and Violence Against Women of Color. *Stanford Law Review* 43: 1241–1299.
Doe, Jane. 2012. Who Benefits from the Sexual Assault Evidence Kit? In *Sexual Assault in Canada*, ed. E. A. Sheehy, 357–388. Ottawa: University of Ottawa Press.
Donnelly, D. A., K. J. Cook, and L. A. Wilson. 1999. Provision and Exclusion: The Dual Face of Services to Battered Women in Three Deep South States. *Violence against Women* 5: 710–741.
Donovan, Roxanne, and Michelle Williams. 2002. Living at the Intersection: The Effects of Racism and Sexism on Black Rape Survivors. *Women & Therapy* 25: 95–105.
Dudley, Rachel. 2012. Toward an Understanding of the 'Medical Plantation' as a Cultural Location of Disability. *Disability Studies Quarterly* 32.
Estrich, Susan. 1987. *Real Rape: How the Legal System Victimizes Women Who Say No*. Cambridge, MA: Harvard University Press.
Harris, Trudier. 1982. *From Mammies to Militants: Domestics in Black American Literature*. Philadelphia: Temple University Press.
Henslin, James, and Mae Biggs. 1971. The Sociology of the Vaginal Exam. In *The Sociology of Sex*, ed. J. Henslin and E. Sagarin, 140–171. New York: Appleton-Century-Crofts.
Hine, Darlene Clark. 1989. Rape and the Inner Lives of Black Women in the Middle West. *Signs* 14: 912–920.
Hlavka, Heather, and Sameena Mulla. 2018. 'That's How She Talks': Animating Text Message Evidence in the Sexual Assault Trial. *Law and Society Review* 52: 401–435.
Hlavka, Heather, and Sameena Mulla. 2020. Thinking Forensically: Law, Medicine and the Nomos of Sexual Violence. In *Research Handbook on Socio-Legal Studies of Medicine and Health*, ed. M. Jacob and A. Kirkland, 232–254. London: Edward Elgar Press.

Hlavka, Heather, and Sameena Mulla. 2021. *Bodies in Evidence: Gender, Race and Science in Sexual Assault Adjudication*. New York: New York University Press.

International Association for Forensic Nurses. 2013. *Atlas of Sexual Violence*. St. Louis: Mosby.

James, Joy. 2016. The Womb of Western Theory: Trauma, Time, Theft and the Captive Maternal. *Carceral Notebooks* 12: 253–296.

James, Joy. 2023. The Captive Maternal is a Function, Not an Identity Marker. *Scalawag*. https://scalawagmagazine.org/2023/04/captive-maternal-joy-james/. Accessed on 20 December 2023.

Kapsalis, Teresa. 1997. *Public Privates: Performing Gynecology from Both Ends of the Speculum*. Durham, NC: Duke University Press.

Kelley, Shamika M. 2023. Post-Sexual Assault Decision Making: Centering Black Women's Experiences. *Feminist Criminology* 18: 133–155.

Ledray, Linda. 1999. *Sexual Assault Nurse Examiner (SANE) Development and Operation Guide*. Washington, DC: U.S. Department of Justice.

Maier, Shana. 2008. 'I Have Heard Terrible Stories...': Rape Victim Advocates' Perceptions of the Revictimization of Rape Victims by the Police and Medical System. *Violence against Women* 14: 786–808.

Mann, Justin. 2019. Dark Matters: On Surveillance of Blackness by Simone Browne (Review). *Palimpsest* 8: 77–79.

McGuire, Danielle. 2017. *At the Dark End of the Street: Black Women, Rape, and Resistance- A New History of the Civil Rights Movement from Rosa Parks to the Rise of Black Power*. New York: Penguin Random House.

Muhammad, Khalil Gibran. 2010. *The Condemnation of Blackness: Race, Crime and the Making of Modern America*. New York and London: Harvard University Press.

Mulla, Sameena. 2023. Intersectionality and Ethnography: Sexual Violence and Racial Subordination in the Courts. In *The Routledge Companion to Intersectionalities*, ed. J. Nash and S. Pinto, 153–160. New York and London: Routledge.

Mulla, Sameena. 2014. *The Violence of Care: Rape Victims, Forensic Nurses, and Sexual Assault Examination*. New York: New York University Press.

Pokorak, Jeffrey J. 2006. Rape as a Badge of Slavery: The Legal History of, and Remedies for, Prosecutorial Race-of-Victim Charging Disparities. *Nevada Law Journal* 7: 1–54.

Potter, Hillary. 2010. 'I don't think a cop has ever asked me if I was OK': Battered Women's Experiences With Police Intervention. In *Female Victims of Crime: Reality Reconsidered*, ed. V. Garcia and J. Clifford, 219–242. Upper Saddle River, NJ: Prentice Hall.

Powell, Amber, Heather Hlavka, and Sameena Mulla. 2017. Intersectionality and Credibility in Child Sexual Assault Trials. *Gender and Society* 31: 457–480.

Powell, Amber, Sameena Mulla, and Heather Hlavka. 2022. Intersectionality in the Courts: Collaborative Feminist Ethnography of Sexual Assault Adjudication. In *Researching Gender-Based Violence: Embodied and Intersectional Approaches*, ed. A. Petillo and H. Hlavka, 159–174. New York: New York University.

Quinlan, Andrea. 2017. *The Technoscientific Witness of Rape*. Toronto: University of Toronto Press.

Richie, Beth. 2012. *Arrested Justice: Black Women, Violence, and America's Prison Nation*. New York: New York University Press.

Ridgeway, Cecilia, and Tamar Krichell-Katz. 2013. Intersecting Cultural Beliefs in Social Relations: Gender, Race, and Class Binds and Freedoms. *Gender & Society* 27: 294–318.

Roberts, Dorothy. 1997. *Killing the Black Body: Race, Reproduction and the Meaning of Liberty*. New York: Vintage Books.

Ruiz, Ashley M., Kaylen Moore, Lynne Woehrle, Penninah Kako, Kelly C. Davis, and Lucy Mkadawire-Valhmu. 2023. Experience of Dehumanizing: Examining Secondary Victimization within the Nurse-Patient Relationship Among African American Women Survivors of Sexual Assault in the Upper Midwest. *Social Science and Medicine* 329. https://doi.org/10.1016/j.socscimed.2023.116029

Sommers, Marilyn, T. M. Zink, J. D. Fargo, R. B. Baker, C. Buschur, D. Z. Shambley-Ebron, and B. S. Fisher. 2008. Forensic Sexual Assault Examination and Genital Injury: Is Skin Color a Source of Health Disparity?". *American Journal of Emergency Medicine* 26: 857–866.

Somerville, Diane. 2004. *Rape and Race in the Nineteenth-Century South*. Chapel Hill, NC: University of North Carolina Press.

Thompson, Mikah. 2021. Just Another Fast Girl: Exploring Slavery's Continued Impact on the Loss of Black Girlhood. *Harvard Journal of Law and Gender* 44: 57–100.

Tynes, Brendane. 2022. 'Sometimes There Just Ain't No Magic in This': Black Women at the Nexus of Gendered Violence and Erasure. In *Researching Gender-Based Violence: Embodied and Intersectional Approaches*, ed. A. Petillo and H. Hlavka, 27–42. New York: New York University Press.

Washington, Harriet. 2001. *Medical Apartheid: The Dark History of Medical Experimentation on Black Americans from Colonial Times to the Present*. New York: Vintage Books.

West, Carolyn M. 2008. Manny, Jezebel, Sapphire, and Their Homegirls: Developing an "Oppositional" Gaze Toward the Images of Black Women. In *Lectures on the Psychology of Women*, 4th ed., ed. J. C. Chrisler, C. Goldern, and P. D. Rozee, 287–299. New York: McGraw-Hill.

Williams, Patricia. 1989. The Obliging Shell: An Informal Essay on Formal Equal Opportunity. *Michigan Law Review* 87: 2128–2151.

# Sleep Medicine Expertise and Sexual Offences: An Unsettled and Unsettling Alliance

*Gethin Rees, Deborah White, and Natalie Wortley*

Following an evening out in London in 2017, Jade McCrossen-Nethercott returned to a friend's house for an after-party, where she eventually fell asleep on a sofa. She woke to find that her clothes had been removed and felt that she had been penetrated. The suspect was still at the other end of the sofa and, when Jade confronted him about what had happened, he said he had thought she was awake. Believing she had

G. Rees (✉)
Newcastle University, Newcastle, UK
e-mail: gethin.rees@newcastle.ac.uk

D. White
Trent University, Peterborough, ON, Canada
e-mail: deborahwhite2@trentu.ca

N. Wortley
Northumbria University, Newcastle Upon Tyne, UK





R. E. Keyse et al. (eds.), *Sexual Violence in Medicine and Psychiatry*, Genders and Sexualities in History,
https://doi.org/10.1007/978-3-032-10800-5_7

been raped, Jade called a friend who was not at the party, who suggested they contact the police.[1]

As part of the police interview (which took place a few weeks after the incident), Jade was asked a series of questions about her sleep behaviour. She reported that she was a very deep sleeper and a heavy snorer and that there had been an incident in the past when she was unable to be roused during a fire alarm. Jade also indicated a history of sleep-talking and sleepwalking. She explained that her partner would recall conversations they had had while she was asleep. Jade explained that her father and grandmother had also displayed sleep behaviours (often referred to as parasomnias), potentially evidencing a hereditary link.

Following disclosure of Jade's police interview, the defence instructed a sleep expert to consider whether Jade could have been in a state of sexsomnia at the relevant time. While the expert did not speak to Jade directly or have any contact with her, the expert's report noted that 'a history of sleepwalking, even if only once, would establish a predisposition to sexsomnia'. Moreover, the expert claimed that the absence of any previous history of sexual behaviour in sleep was not determinative, as the event in question could be the first time that Jade's parasomnia had manifested in a sexual manner.

In response to a defence request to comment specifically on how Jade would have presented during an episode of sexsomnia, the expert noted that 'her behaviour would have been of someone actively engaging in sexual activity, with eyes open and showing pleasure'. Based upon this report, and given that the suspect maintained he had reasonably believed Jade to be consenting, the Crown Prosecution Service (CPS) informed Jade that they no longer felt there was a realistic prospect of conviction and had decided to stop the case.

The use of sleep medicine expertise in the criminal justice system has long been controversial. Sleep expert evidence has been deployed on a number of occasions in support of claims that defendants were experiencing episodes of sexsomnia at the time of their alleged offences but this appears to be the first time that such expertise has been mobilised to attack the credibility of a complainant. This is a significant (and, given the controversy, a potentially troubling) development. In this chapter we will

[1] The case details are taken from the BBC documentary *Sexsomnia: Case Closed*, which can be viewed here: https://www.bbc.co.uk/programmes/p0cyrmzv#:~:text=When%20unexpected%20sleepwalking%20claims%20turn,one%20woman's%20battle%20for%20justice.

discuss the debate concerning the legitimacy of the knowledge and practices that underpin sleep medicine expertise and its applicability in forensic contexts. We will show that the threshold for a diagnosis of parasomnia is very low and explore how recent developments in sleep medicine have made it increasingly difficult to challenge claims around parasomnias and related defences. Finally, we will explore whether existing criminal justice rules and procedures could be invoked to ensure fairness to those harmed.

## 1 Background

### *1.1 Parasomnias and Sexsomnia*

Sexsomnia is a form of Non-REM parasomnia, like sleepwalking, sleep-talking or sleep-eating. It occurs when a person is in deep sleep (technically referred to as Slow-Wave Sleep). The sleeper might transition to a lighter level of sleep, but without being fully conscious (i.e. they are still asleep). While in this state a person can perform a range of activities without having any recollection of them. At its simplest, for a parasomnia to be diagnosed at least two of the following three factors will ordinarily be present: predisposing; priming; and/or precipitating (triggering) factors (Pressman 2007; Rees and White 2022). Predisposing factors relate to a genetic/family history of parasomnias; priming factors are contextual and could be environmental or lifestyle-related (e.g. overweight, diet) and/or a known-history of disturbed sleep behaviours (e.g. a personal history of sleepwalking); finally, triggering factors are immediate events that bring a person from the deeper level of sleep to the lighter level (e.g. contact with a bed partner, or light/sound in the room). If at least two factors can be identified, then a night-time activity can be identified as a parasomnia (American Academy of Sleep Medicine (AASM) 2014). As its name suggests, the term 'sexsomnia' signifies sleep-based activities involving sexual behaviours (e.g., masturbation, moaning and/or engaging in sexual intercourse) (AASM 2014).

### *1.2 The Legal Context*

Medical sleep expertise has a long tradition within the criminal courtroom. Since at least the mid-nineteenth century, medical experts are known to have provided testimony on behalf of defendants claiming to have been asleep at the time of their alleged criminal conduct (Eigen

2003; Melechi 2003). It is generally accepted that, where an offence requires proof of a positive act, a defendant will only be liable if the prosecution can prove their conduct was voluntary. While the label of 'voluntariness' and its meaning are contested by some legal academics, for our purposes it is sufficient to note that the actions of a person who is sleepwalking are involuntary, notwithstanding that their outward movements may appear to be coordinated. Accordingly, save where involuntariness is caused by D's[2] own prior fault (as discussed below), they cannot be guilty of an offence because their lack of capacity to control their actions negates criminal responsibility.

### *1.2.1 Insane and Non-insane Automatism*

The rule that physical involuntariness precludes criminal responsibility poses two key dilemmas for the criminal law. First, there are examples of individuals causing serious harm by actions over which they had no conscious control (e.g. *R v Kemp* 1957; *R v Sullivan* 1984; *R v Burgess* 1991). Since the aims of the criminal law include both the prevention of conduct that threatens substantial harm to individual or public interests and the subjection to public control of those who are disposed to commit crimes (American Law Institute 1962; Criminal Procedure Rules 2020), fairness to individuals who lack the capacity to control their actions has to be balanced against the need to protect the public. Secondly, an individual may be responsible for inducing the lack of capacity which caused them to engage in acts that would ordinarily amount to a criminal offence (e.g. by voluntarily ingesting alcohol or failing to take prescribed medication). The fault inherent in this prior conduct may mean that it is both appropriate and necessary for criminal liability to attach despite their lack of control at the time of the alleged offence.

As to the first of these dilemmas, the common law seeks to strike an appropriate balance by distinguishing between states of automatism that result from an external cause (and which it assumes are therefore unlikely to recur), and those that result from an internal condition. The former is labelled 'sane automatism' (or 'non-insane automatism') and, if successfully pleaded, results in acquittal. The latter is known as 'insane automatism' (more commonly, 'insanity') and a successful plea results in

[2] D here is legal nomenclature for Defendant.

the special verdict of 'not guilty by reason of insanity' ('NGBRI') (Criminal Procedure (Insanity) Act 1964, s.1). While a court ordinarily has no power to impose any sanction or restrictions upon someone who has been acquitted of an offence, a verdict of NGBRI requires the judge to make a hospital order (with or without a restriction order), a supervision order, or an absolute discharge.[3] A hospital order constitutes a serious deprivation of a person's liberty and may only be made if there is expert psychiatric evidence that the defendant has a mental disorder that warrants their compulsory detention in a hospital for treatment (Mental Health Act 1983, s.37). In addition, a variety of ancillary orders and provisions that apply to convicted offenders also apply to offenders who are found not guilty by reason of insanity, including the obligation to comply with notification requirements under the Sexual Offences Act (2003), where applicable.[4]

The law provides that where a state of automatism was caused by an external factor, the defendant may plead (sane) automatism but where there is no external factor, the appropriate plea is one of insanity and the controversial *M'Naghten* Rules apply (*M'Naghten's Case,* 1843).[5] This 'can give rise to apparently strange results at the margin' (*R v C* 2013, 20). In *R v Quick* (1973), for example, a nurse took his prescribed insulin but then failed to eat, resulting in a hypoglycaemic episode during which he attacked a patient. The Court of Appeal held that the taking of insulin was an external factor and the defendant ought to have been permitted to rely on the defence of automatism at his trial. Conversely, in *R v Hennessy,* (1989), the defendant failed to take his prescribed dose of insulin and, while suffering from hyperglycaemia, took a motor vehicle without the consent of the owner. The Court of Appeal held that the trial judge had been correct to rule that the only available defence was one of insanity. Hennessy's condition had been caused by his diabetes; the stress, anxiety and depression that caused him to forget his insulin were 'not ... in themselves, separately or together external factors of the kind capable in law

[3] Criminal Procedure (Insanity) Act (1964, s.5A). A restriction order places certain limitations upon the power to discharge a patient from hospital.

[4] Commonly known as 'the Sex Offenders' Register'.

[5] The *M'Naghten* Rules state that every person is presumed to be sane but that a defence of insanity will be available if it is proved that the defendant was labouring under a defect of reason from a disease of the mind such that they either did not know the nature and quality of the act or did not know that it was wrong.

of causing or contributing to a state of [sane] automatism' (*R v Hennessy* 1989, 294).

The application of the external/internal factor test similarly makes little medical sense in the context of parasomnias (Law Commission 2013, 5.58). Early cases suggested that a person who committed what would otherwise be a crime while asleep could rely on (sane) automatism (*R v Tolson* 1889, 187; *Bratty v A-G for Northern Ireland* 1963, 409). However, in *R v Burgess* (1991), the Court of Appeal held that expert evidence that the defendant had been sleepwalking when they committed an act of serious violence could only support a defence of insanity. The defendant's 'state of somnambulism' was 'an abnormality or disorder, albeit transitory, due to an internal factor …' (*R v Burgess* 1991, 101). The risk of recurrence was an additional reason for categorising the condition as a 'disease of the mind' (*R v Burgess* 1991, 99). But refusing to allow someone who claims to suffer from parasomnia to avail themselves of an automatism defence is problematic, as it means that invoking involuntariness exposes them to the stigma of being labelled 'insane' despite sleep being a 'normal condition' (*Parks v R* 1992).

Notwithstanding the precedent of *R v Burgess* (1991), there is evidence that courts of first instance have sometimes taken a more inclusionary approach to the automatism defence in the context of parasomnias and defendants have been permitted to plead (sane) automatism where medical evidence of sleepwalking was available.[6] In *R v Bilton* (2005) (see also Ebrahim 2006), the defendant was charged with rape and claimed to have been sleepwalking at the time. He was acquitted (rather than being found NGBRI), indicating that the trial judge left the defence of automatism to the jury despite the apparent lack of any external factor.[7] Other jurisdictions have similarly taken a broad approach to the relevance of parasomnias and categorised them as forms of sane automatism on the ground that 'the distinction between internal and external causes is blurred during sleep' (*Parks v R* 1992).[8] As explained above and explored further below, predisposing and priming factors are relevant when diagnosing sleep disorders but precipitating (i.e. external) factors may also

[6] Transcripts of trials are not published in England and Wales so we are largely dependent on reporting of cases in the press.

[7] See also *R v Davies* (unreported) (*The Times* 11 February 2006); cf. *R v Kelly* (unreported) (*The Guardian* 20 August 2019).

[8] See also *Rabey v R* (1980).

contribute to an episode of parasomnia. Sleepwalking may therefore occur with or without an external trigger.

### *1.2.2 Prior Fault and Liability*

As to the second dilemma to which we refer above, the question is whether a defendant should be considered criminally culpable if they were responsible for bringing about their lack of capacity. A driver who falls asleep at the wheel is blameworthy because there was a point at which they chose to carry on driving despite recognising that they were tired. Similarly, if it could be shown that the consumption of alcohol was a trigger for sleepwalking in a particular case, the defendant could be said to be responsible in that they chose to consume the alcohol that caused them later to lack the ability to control their bodily movements.

The doctrine of prior fault precludes a defendant from invoking a defence of automatism if their condition was self-induced or if incapacity 'could have been reasonably foreseen as a result of either doing, or omitting to do something as, for example, taking alcohol against medical advice after using certain prescribed drugs or failing to have regular meals while taking insulin' (*R v Quick* 1973). The prior fault principle also applies in cases of voluntary intoxication to prevent offenders from escaping liability by claiming that they were so intoxicated that they failed to form the mental element required by the definition of the offence charged. The appellate courts have repeatedly emphasised that 'a drunken intent is nevertheless an intent' (*R v Sheehan & Moore* 1975) and 'in the great majority of cases of alleged sexual assault, or of comparable sexual crimes ... the mind will have gone with the touching, penetration or other prohibited act, albeit in some cases a drunken mind' (*R v Heard* 2007). Where, exceptionally, the jury cannot be sure that a voluntarily intoxicated defendant acted with *mens rea* but they are satisfied the defendant would have foreseen the risk of their actions if they had been sober, they are entitled to be acquitted of a crime of specific intent but remain liable to be convicted of a lesser, basic intent offence.[9]

[9] Basic intent offences are, generally, offences that can be committed either intentionally or recklessly. For these crimes, the act of voluntarily consuming intoxicants is deemed to satisfy the element of recklessness so as to enable courts to ascribe criminal liability (*DPP v Majewski* 1977). All the main offences under the Sexual Offences Act 2003, including rape and sexual assault, are crimes of basic intent (*R v Heard* 2007).

Where a lack of capacity has concurrent or consecutive causes, one of which may include intoxication, the position is less clear, and it is difficult to discern a coherent approach. However, the basis of the intoxication rules is that 'where a man of his own volition takes a substance which causes him to cast off the restraints of reason and conscience, no wrong is done to him by holding him answerable criminally for any injury he may do while in that condition' (*DPP v Majewski* 1977). Accordingly, where a defendant claims to have been 'sleepwalking' due to the external factor of alcohol consumption, the intoxication rules will apply if D was still intoxicated at the relevant time (Child et al. 2020). The decision in *R v Taj* (2018) suggests that the intoxication rules may also encompass a failure to form *mens rea* 'immediately and proximately consequent upon earlier drink or drug-taking, so that even though the person concerned is not drunk or intoxicated at the time, the short-term effects can be shown to have triggered subsequent episodes of *e.g.* paranoia'.

### *1.3 Expert Evidence*

In a case in which a defendant claims to have been sleepwalking when committing an alleged offence, medical evidence will always be required. Such evidence will first need to support the presence of parasomnia. Secondly, the defendant will typically hope that such evidence will confirm the existence of an external trigger as a contributing factor, as this will facilitate a claim of automatism which will result in an acquittal if pleaded successfully. If there is no evidence of an external factor, a decision will need to be taken as to whether to plead insanity. In some cases, and for some defendants, the prospect of criminal conviction may be preferable to risking indefinite detention in hospital and the stigma of the insanity label, though this may depend upon the nature and length of the sentence that is likely to follow a plea or finding of guilt (Law Commission 2013, 8.54).

#### *1.3.1 A Forensic Sleep Medicine Controversy*

While many of the early reported cases involving parasomnias, in particular sleepwalking, related to murder, during the 1990s case histories of sexual offence trials increasingly began to appear in the forensic medical literature. At that time there was a strong consensus among the sleep medicine community about what constituted the triggers for sleepwalking, which fed neatly into the binary legal discourses required (i.e. whether the cause of the parasomnia was internal or external and whether a defence of insanity or automatism applied). This consensus was shattered in 2007, however, following the publication of a case report in the *Journal of Clinical Forensic Medicine* (Ebrahim 2006), in which the author drew attention to a sexsomnia trial in which the suspect had consumed alcohol before going to sleep. In preparing for this case, the respective experts instructed by the prosecution (Fenwick) and the defence (Ebrahim) worked together to investigate the suspect's potential sleep condition. Using the traditional clinical tests for sleep disorders, polysomnography (PSG),[10] Ebrahim and Fenwick developed a three night protocol to ascertain whether there was any evidence that the accused had a sleep disorder. This included an acclimatisation night (getting the sleeper used to the laboratory environment), a baseline night to assess the patient's underlying sleep architecture and finally a challenge night, where triggering factors might be added and their impact assessed. In this case, as the suspect had been intoxicated before the criminal act, alcohol was used as the trigger.

Ebrahim reported that while the baseline night did provide evidence that the suspect had a breathing disorder that could produce parasomnias, the PSG also showed evidence of disturbances within sleep following the alcohol trigger (or 'alcohol challenge') on the third night, suggesting that alcohol could also have played a role. If alcohol did constitute a trigger for the parasomnia, then it would constitute an external cause and support a defence of non-insane automatism. To this end, Ebrahim and Fenwick produced a joint report for the court with the outcome of their findings and, notwithstanding the law on prior fault discussed above, the accused was reportedly acquitted.

Following the publication of this article, Pressman and colleagues (Pressman et al. 2007a; see also Pressman et al. 2007b) wrote a letter to the editors of the *Journal of Forensic and Legal Medicine* robustly challenging Ebrahim and Fenwick's methodology. The authors argued that alcohol is not a trigger for parasomnias and that polysomnography is an inappropriate tool for forensic purposes, as PSG evidence is not

[10] Polysomnography is an investigation normally conducted in a sleep clinic, where a person's brain waves while asleep are electronically recorded via an electroencephalogram (EEG), their muscle tone and movement recorded via electromyogram (EMG), eye-movement recorded via electrooculogram (EOG) and heart rate recorded by electrocardiogram (EGG) (Ebrahim et al., 2005).

sufficiently objective or precise to justify its use in a forensic context. In particular, they argued that there is no means of determining whether a person was in a parasomnia state at the time of a criminal act and polysomnographic evidence might give the impression that sleep experts can be more definitive about the accused's state of mind/consciousness at the time of the criminal act than is, in fact, possible. Moreover, they contended that Ebrahim and Fenwick had invented a test, namely the alcohol challenge that had no basis in medical knowledge or practice.

For the next decade the sleep medicine community was involved in a heated controversy, split between those who supported Ebrahim and Fenwick and considered alcohol to be a trigger factor for parasomnias, and the supporters of Pressman and colleagues, who strenuously argued that it was not.[11] One key plank of Pressman and colleagues' critique related to the utility of PSG as a forensic tool and whether there were any potential indicators that signify conditions that were more likely to produce a parasomnia (for instance, when intoxicated, as Ebrahim and Fenwick suggested). While it was generally accepted that full-blown parasomnias were unlikely to manifest in the clinical environment, predominantly due to the variety of factors that need to be present to instigate a behaviour, some sleep experts considered there to be particular signs on the PSG recording that are diagnostic, or at least indicative of an underlying parasomnia. For instance, two factors originally identified by Ebrahim et al. (2005) concerned a high rate of arousals during Slow Wave Sleep, and a lower quantity of deep sleep in the early stages of the sleep cycle. An arousal in this context refers to an abrupt jump from Slow-Wave Sleep to a lighter level (technically referred to as stages 1, 2, or even REM sleep) without traversing the other stages, which is identified as a violent peak on the polysomnographic recording. This arousal might be accompanied by a physical reaction, which would also then be recorded on video camera. Ebrahim and colleagues stated that a high rate of such arousals is indicative of a tendency towards sleepwalking (Ebrahim et al. 2005); with Ebrahim going further and noting in the case report that instigated the controversy that more than 15 arousals in a single night's sleep would be considered excessive (Ebrahim and Fenwick 2007). Given these arousals,

[11] There is not the space to explore fully the details of the controversy in this chapter and we will concentrate solely on the debates around the role of PSG here. For summaries and reviews of the wider controversy, especially concerning the role of alcohol intoxication as a trigger for parasomnia, see Jackson et al. (2015) and Rees and White (2022).

it also follows that those with less overall time in Slow Wave Sleep during the early stages of sleep, when evaluated with age and sex comparators, is also indicative of an underlying parasomnia (Ebrahim et al. 2005).

Ebrahim and colleagues' claims around the significance of arousals in the early part of sleep were heavily contested by Pressman and colleagues. They argued that while the relationship between higher rates of arousals and sleepwalking is statistically significant, it has not been found to be clinically significant and, moreover, is not specifically diagnostic for parasomnia, as high rates of arousals have also been found in those with sleep apnoea and periodic leg movement (Pressman et al. 2007b). Similarly, Ebrahim's assertion that 15 arousals in the early part of sleep is excessive is not derived from the specific sleepwalking literature. A similar figure (15) for arousals appears in the scientific literature in relation to an apnoea/hypopnea index but, again, this relates to sleep apnoea and not sleepwalking. On this basis, Pressman and colleagues argued that the technical indicators, which Ebrahim and colleagues considered to be indicative (if not diagnostic) of parasomnias, were insufficiently sensitive, specific or based in the scientific literature to be taken seriously and ought not to be used in criminal justice contexts. A similar claim was made in relation to Ebrahim's other indicator, the low overall quantity of Slow-Wave Sleep, with Gaudreau and colleagues explaining that:

> [g]iven the likelihood that results of our study could be used in medico-legal settings, it is worth noting that the presence or absence of a decrease of SWA [Slow Wave Activity] early in the night and of awakenings from SWS [Slow Wave Sleep] in a given individual does not conclusively establish or refute a tendency toward sleepwalking. (Gaudreau et al. 2000, 4–5)

While the next ten years was spent further exploring technical artefacts and conducting investigations that might be efficacious in helping identify parasomnias, their usage continued to be undermined by the criticism that they lacked sensitivity or specificity, especially in forensic contexts.

In 2013, both the *Diagnostic and Statistical Manual of Mental Disorders 5* (DSM-5 2013) and the *International Classification of Sleep Disorders 3* (AASM 2014) were updated. The former now states that, '[i]n the absence of actually capturing an event during a polysomnographic recording, there are no polysomnographic features that can serve as a marker for sleepwalking' (APA 2013, 402). The manual does acknowledge that polysomnography can be useful for supporting clinical decisions, '[o]n rare occasions… by documenting arousals from slow wave sleep accompanied by behaviours typical of confusional arousals' (AASM 2014, 236). However, it reiterates that these behaviours are often rare in the laboratory and, if PSG is to be used, '[t]ime-synchronized video-polysomnographic (vPSG) is essential' (AASM 2014, 236), as this will capture both physical manifestations and the brain wave recording. Importantly, this emphasises that the presence of behaviour within the clinic that is diagnostic of sleepwalking and, by extension, the absence of either a full-blown physical manifestation of a sleepwalking behaviour or any indications of technical phenomena on the recordings (for instance, arousals), should not be counted as contra-indications to the person being a sleepwalker. In addition, the DSM categorises alcoholic blackout as involving a different mental state to sleepwalking.

### 1.3.2 *Whither Forensic Sleep Medicine Expertise?*

In the absence of technical evidence to help support a diagnosis the expert is left with medical history. Following the publication of both the DSM-5 and ICSD3, Idzikowski published an essay setting out the responsibilities of the sleep clinician/expert particularly with respect to sexual behaviours in sleep (Idzikowski 2014). He returned to classic sleep diagnostic guidance produced in 1974 to explain how a clinician/sleep expert should go about assessing a potential sexsomnia case. Idzikowski's summary of these earlier guidelines emphasised:

(1) the importance of ascertaining whether there is any personal and/or familial history of sleepwalking, both of which could be corroborated by third parties;
(2) that in relation to the conduct in question, the person should have slept for long enough to have entered the Slow Wave Sleep state, but not so long that they should be in REM sleep (so approximately within two to three hours or sleeping) and that sleep should have been particularly deep due to a specific factor, for instance stress, fatigue or fever;
(3) that the sexsomnia behaviour that is claimed should be short (noted by Idzikowski as between a few and 30 minutes) and the victim should be nearby;
(4) on awakening, the patient/defendant should have no recollection of their actions and should be confused.

Taking these factors into consideration, alongside the history of the specific act, especially any predisposing, priming and precipitating factors, the sleep expert should be able to assess whether the individual has an underlying sleep condition or, in a forensic context, whether a particular act was potentially the result of a sleep condition.

While these guidelines do require a modicum of expert knowledge (e.g. awareness of how long it takes someone to enter Slow Wave Sleep and the length of time they are likely to remain in that state), much of the information necessary to make a diagnosis of parasomnia is non-scientific. Perhaps even more problematically, consideration of whether someone has a personal or familial history of sleepwalking is predominantly based on self-disclosure, and there is therefore a risk that this may rely on assumptions about post-sleep behaviours. For instance, actions that might be labelled by members of the public as 'sleepwalking' may be performed for a range of other reasons (e.g. alcoholic blackout; undiagnosed epilepsy; or, diabetes). As Pressman (2013) noted, if a person who is intoxicated subsequently performs movements after going to bed, their actions may be labelled by those around them as sleepwalking when they are in fact acting during an alcoholic blackout. If subsequently asked whether they have experienced sleepwalking in the past, they may categorically answer in the affirmative, because 'sleepwalking' is the everyday label that has been attached to their activities after going to bed. While the classic guidelines may be helpful in a clinical context given the relatively low stakes relating to a false diagnosis of parasomnia, they are problematic as a tool for diagnosing or labelling a particular activity as the product of a parasomnia in the forensic context, where a miscarriage of justice may ensue from a false diagnosis.

In demonstrating the flaws inherent in the clinical tools used to investigate sleepwalking, Pressman et al. have shown that sleep medicine can only be of limited assistance to the trier of fact in criminal proceedings. In the absence of a full-blown parasomnia manifesting within a clinical investigation, there is no evidence that a person is (or is not) a sleepwalker. Even if someone has a history of sleepwalking, there is uncertainty as to whether their mental state is consistent with a parasomnia or whether post-bed activities are attributable to another cause. In addition, the controversy made clear that even with a clinically diagnosed parasomnia, a sleep expert cannot ascertain with certainty whether a person was sleepwalking at the time of the alleged event, although, following classic diagnostic guidelines, and with particular information (for instance, the period of time for which the person had been asleep) they can provide some conclusions as to the likelihood that their actions were consistent with a parasomnia.

This low-bar of entry for a parasomnia diagnosis to enter is further problematic if a criminal accused draws upon the potential for the victim-survivor to have been in a sleepwalking state in an effort to support a defence of reasonable belief in consent. Given our account of the recent history of forensic sleep medicine, it is perhaps unsurprising that the sleep expert in Jade's case did not feel it necessary to clinically investigate Jade to prepare their report. The disclosures made by Jade during the police interview provided both a personal history of sleep-talking and sleepwalking, as well as a family history and therefore meet two of the classic guideline's criteria. It is not clear whether the sleep expert was aware of how long Jade had been asleep at the time that the sexual assault occurred (and so whether a parasomnia could have been ruled out) and, given that alcohol-intoxication is deemed to be a different state of mind to sleepwalking following the ICSD3 and DSM-5, there perhaps should have been some discussion of whether alcohol itself may have negated sexsomnia. Finally, it seems noteworthy that the expert expressed that Jade's 'behaviour would have been of someone actively engaging in sexual activity, with eyes open and showing pleasure', when much of the literature on parasomnias and sexual behaviours emphasises the 'glassy-eyed stare' of the sleepwalker. For instance, the ICSD3 states: 'The eyes are usually open during an episode and, not uncommonly, are wide open with a confused "glassy" stare' (AASM 2014, 230). In fact, many bed partners often acknowledge that their partner is in a sexsomnia episode because of the confused, glassy look (Mangan 2001), which sounds significantly different to 'showing pleasure'. Ultimately, while the expert evidence in this case, as we understand it,[12] is not without problems, it is consistent with the process of expert decision-making set out in the classic guidelines. As a result, it is alarmingly difficult for the prosecution to undermine or challenge a claim of sleepwalking. As Jade's case shows, prosecutors may also struggle to negate a defence claim that the survivor of a sexual assault acted in a state of sexsomnia where that claim is supported by expert evidence. This is, at least in part, a consequence of the allocation

[12] And aware we have not reviewed the expert report ourselves.

of the burden of proof in criminal cases and it is to this issue that we now turn.

## 2 Criminal Justice Processing in Parasomnia/Sexsomnia Cases

### *2.1 Burden of Proof and Charging Decisions*

The claim made by the accused in Jade's case was in one sense analogous to a sane automatism plea. An allegation of rape requires the prosecution to make the jury sure of the following: (1) that the defendant intentionally penetrated the vagina, anus or mouth of the complainant; (2) the complainant was not consenting at the time; and (3) the defendant did not reasonably believe the complainant was consenting (Sexual Offences Act 2003, s.1). Since the prosecution bears the legal burden of proving all three elements, where it is claimed that the complainant was suffering from sexsomnia there is theoretically no requirement for a defendant to produce medical evidence to support this contention. However, it seems highly unlikely that a jury would regard a mere assertion by a defendant as giving rise to reasonable doubt about guilt—and it is inconceivable that the prosecution would accept it and offer no evidence against the defendant. Thus, in Jade's case, the defence requested an expert report, presumably in the hope that this would support their client's case. The prosecution would then have to make the jury sure that Jade was not in a sexsomnia state at the time in order to prove the defendant did not reasonably believe she was consenting.

In deciding whether there is sufficient evidence to charge a suspect with an offence, Crown Prosecutors must apply the two-stage 'Full Code Test' laid down in the Code for Crown Prosecutors (Director of Public Prosecutions, 2018). First, is there sufficient credible, reliable and admissible evidence to provide a 'realistic prospect of conviction' (Director of Public Prosecutions 2018, 4.6). In assessing the sufficiency of evidence, a prosecutor must consider any defence that has been put forward and any other information upon which the suspect may rely and must determine whether it is more likely than not that a tribunal of fact would convict (Director of Public Prosecutions 2018, 4.6–4.8). If the evidential threshold for prosecution is met, consideration must then be given to whether a prosecution is required in the public interest (Director of Public Prosecutions 2018, 4.9). To reach a Code-compliant decision at the evidential stage, prosecutors must 'carefully consider all relevant evidence from an informed position', which requires 'a comprehensive understanding of … the dynamics of the offence including the tactics deployed by offenders as well as the complexities of rape and victim behaviours' (Director of Public Prosecutions, 2020). As separate guidance makes clear, 'rape myths and stereotypes should play no part' in prosecutorial decision making (Crown Prosecution Service 2021).

We do not know the full extent of the evidence that was available in Jade's case but we know she had given her account during a video recorded interview.[13] Such interviews should be carried out in accordance with national guidance (Ministry of Justice 2022), which recommends a four-stage approach, comprising:

(1) Rapport;
(2) Free-narrative account;
(3) Topic division, followed by clarification and development of the account, systematic introduction and probing of any wider investigative material that may be important to the investigation;
(4) Closure.

Jade appears to have given a clear and coherent account of what happened insofar as she could remember the events. We also know that the defendant made no comment when interviewed, although it appears to be accepted that, when Jade awoke and realised she had been penetrated, the suspect said 'I thought you were awake'. This looks like an admission that sexual intercourse had taken place, although no explanation was put forward by the suspect at that stage as to why he claimed that he thought Jade was awake. The totality of the evidence would appear to meet the evidential threshold and the suspect was indeed charged with rape.

However, Crown Prosecutors are under a duty to continually review cases and to consider any change in circumstances, including what becomes known of the defence case (Director of Public Prosecutions

[13] Complainants in cases involving sexual offences are automatically entitled to special measures to support them to give their best evidence (Youth Justice and Criminal Evidence Act 1999, s.17(4)). These measures include the use of video recorded interviews as the witness's evidence-in-chief. Such interviews should be carried out in accordance with national guidance (Ministry of Justice 2022).

2018, 3.6). They should seek to rectify evidential weaknesses where possible but 'should quickly stop cases which do not meet the evidential stage of the Full Code Test' (Director of Public Prosecutions 2018, 3.4). When the defence served their expert report in Jade's case, the prosecutor was required to consider it and to decide whether the evidential threshold was still met. Since this decision required consideration of whether there was sufficient credible, reliable and admissible evidence, the prosecution ought to have had regard to whether the expert had complied with rules governing the admissibility and reliability of expert evidence.

### 2.2 *Admissibility of Expert Evidence*

At common law, the following factors apply when the admissibility of expert evidence falls to be determined:

(1) The evidence must be relevant to a matter in issue in the proceedings;
(2) it must be necessary to furnish the court with information that is likely to be outside the experience and knowledge of the judge or jury (known as the 'assistance' requirement) (*R v Turner* 1975);
(3) the individual seeking to provide the evidence must be an expert in the relevant field (the 'competence' or 'relevant expertise' requirement) (*R v Silverlock* 1894; Criminal Procedure Rules 2020, r.19.2(a)(ii));
(4) the expert must be able to provide objective and unbiased evidence on matters within their field of expertise (the 'impartiality' requirement) (*R v Stubbs* 2006; Criminal Procedure Rules 2020, r.19.2(a)(i));
(5) the evidence must be sufficiently reliable to be admitted (the 'evidentiary reliability' requirement) (*R v Dlugosz* 2013).

In addition, recent case law has confirmed that it is not sufficient for an expert to make generalised statements about a particular mental disorder and its potential effects on an individual's behaviour or actions. The expert's opinion must be 'tethered to the evidence about the circumstances of the incident' (*R v Jacobs* 2023).

The Criminal Practice Directions 2023 (CPD)[14] list a series of factors the court may take into account in determining the reliability of expert evidence, particularly scientific expert opinion. The following are particularly relevant to Jade's case: the validity of the methodology employed by the expert (CPD 2023, 7.1.2(b)); if the expert's opinion relies on an inference from any findings, whether the opinion properly explains how safe or unsafe the inference is (CPD 2023, 7.1.2(c)); the extent to which any material upon which the expert's opinion is based has been reviewed by others with relevant expertise (for instance, in peer-reviewed publications), and the views of those others on that material (CPD 2023, 7.1.2(e)); the completeness of the information which was available to the expert, and whether the expert took account of all relevant information in arriving at the opinion (including information as to the context of any facts to which the opinion relates) (CPD 2023, 7.1.2(g)); if there is a range of expert opinion, to specify where within that range the expert's own opinion lies and whether the expert's preference has been properly explained (CPD 2023, 7.1.2(h)); whether the expert methods followed established practice in the field and, if they did not, whether the reason for the diversions has been properly explained (CPD 2023, 7.1.2(i)).

In addition, the CPD warn that the court must be astute to identify potential flaws in expert opinion which detract from its reliability, such as: being based on a hypothesis which has not been subjected to sufficient scrutiny (including, where appropriate, experimental or other testing), or which has failed to stand up to scrutiny (CPD 2023, 7.1.3(a)); being based on an unjustifiable assumption (CPD 2023, 7.1.3(b)); relying on an examination, technique, method or process which was not properly carried out or applied (CPD 2023, 7.1.3(d)); and relying on an inference or conclusion which has not been properly reached (CPD 2023, 7.1.3(e)). In order to enable the reliability of expert evidence to be properly assessed, experts are required to disclose 'all potentially relevant information' (CPD 2023, 7.1.4).

Here, the defence expert's report ought therefore to have explained that there is a lack of established practice when it comes to diagnosing sexsomnia (CPD 2023, 7.1.2(i)). The expert should nevertheless have set out the methodology they employed (CPD 2023, 7.1.2(b)) in forming

[14] Although the version of the Criminal Practice Directions that was in force at the time of Jade's case was the CPD 2020, the directions relating to expert evidence are substantively unchanged in the 2023 iteration of the CPD.

their opinion that Jade may have been experiencing a first episode of sexsomnia. The expert was under a duty to identify any material upon which their opinion was based, such as research papers, and to disclose that other experts have contrary views about that material (CPD 2023, 7.1.2(e), 7.1.2(h) and 7.1.4). In relation to the expert's opinion that, if acting in a state of sexsomnia, Jade would have presented as actively engaging in—and enjoying—sexual activity, the expert was under a duty to point out literature to the contrary, including the ICSD. They should also have outlined any limitations upon their evidence (CPD 2023, 7.1.2(g)), such as the fact that they did not speak to Jade directly, obtain corroborating evidence of her familial/personal sleepwalking history from others and nor did they have access to her medical records (CPD 2023, 7.1.2(e)).

We are reliant on the summary of the defence expert's report in the BBC documentary so we cannot know whether or how it addressed the requirements of the CPD. However, if it had revealed that there were two diametrically opposed schools of thought as to the criteria for diagnosing sexsomnia, the role of alcohol as a trigger, and the extent to which sleep medicine is capable of being used in a forensic context, it seems unlikely the prosecution would have discontinued the case. The position would then have been analogous to a claim of sexsomnia by a defendant, as the same burden and standard of proof applies, in respect of which CPS Guidance indicates the matter should be left to the jury to determine. Indeed, if the prosecution had been made aware of the nature and extent of the controversy, they could have sought to instruct an expert from the opposing side of the debate to ensure the issues could be aired in full. One difficulty, however, with the proposition that opposing expert views should be left to the jury is that it relies on advocates being willing and able to explore the issues in cross-examination. A study carried out one year after the reliability criteria were introduced in England and Wales revealed a lack of awareness on the part of practitioners as to the existence of the criteria and a disinclination to challenge perceived expertise (Davies and Piasecki 2016). There has been a dearth of case law since that time, so it is unclear whether—and to what extent—this has changed.

## 3 What Might Have Happened?

Let us now consider what Jade's case might have looked like in a system in which experts complied with all of their duties, the prosecution was mindful of its own guidance, and the ultimate arbiters of fact were permitted to perform their role. First, it is unlikely that the interviewing officer would ask Jade questions concerning her sleep habits, given that police officers lack expertise in sleep medicine, they cannot know whether such questions are appropriate or necessary. In light of the suspect's assertion that he thought Jade was awake, the defence might nevertheless have instructed an expert to consider whether Jade might have been in a state of sexsomnia at the relevant time. Before forming an opinion, the expert would first obtain a full account from the defendant and, applying the classic diagnostic guidelines, ascertain whether the defendant's claim was feasible having regard to the length of time Jade was asleep, the duration of the sexual activity and his description of Jade's presentation at the time. If these ruled out sexsomnia, the expert would prepare an unfavourable report. If sexsomnia was not ruled out (which seems likely given the low bar for a diagnosis of parasomnia), the expert might endeavour to speak with Jade—and possibly other family members and/or previous bed partners—and potentially seek her permission to access her medical records to establish the nature and extent of any history of parasomnia. On the basis of all available information, the expert would form an opinion as to whether it was possible that Jade may have been suffering from sexsomnia and, if so, would set out the basis for that opinion. All caveats and limitations would be set out in the expert's report, such as the fact that Jade had not previously experienced such an episode and the significance of such limitations for the strength of the expert's opinion would be explained. The prosecution would then instruct their own expert to evaluate the defence expert's opinion and form their own conclusions on the available material, making further enquiries as necessary. The experts would meet and produce a report setting out the matters on which they agreed and the matters on which they disagreed and the reasons why.

Assuming the defendant maintained a not guilty plea and the case proceeded to trial, Jade's pre-recorded interview would be played to the jury, having been edited to remove any irrelevant questions and answers about her sleep history so as to avoid risking the jury making unwarranted assumptions based upon their preconceptions about sleepwalking. Any questions about possible prior episodes of sexsomnia would likely be prohibited as they would constitute questions about previous sexual behaviour, which are generally prohibited (Youth Justice and Criminal Evidence Act 1999, s.41).[15] The court would do what it could to mitigate the re-traumatising properties of the adversarial system, including arranging pre-recorded cross examination in advance of the trial so there would be no need for Jade to attend court (Youth Justice and Criminal Evidence Act 1999, s.28). After Jade's evidence and that of any other prosecution witnesses (such as the friend to whom she made an immediate complaint), the defendant would be invited to testify. Should he decline to do so, the jury would be invited to draw an adverse inference from that failure (Criminal Justice and Public Order Act 1994, s.35).[16] If he were to testify and give a full account of what he claimed happened, including the reasons he believed Jade to be consenting, an inference could still be drawn against him due to his failure to mention those 'facts' when interviewed by the police (Criminal Justice and Public order Act 1994, s.34).[17]

If the expert evidence was not agreed between the parties (as seems likely given the divergence of views between sleep experts on various topics), both the prosecution expert and the defence expert would give evidence. They would be asked to explain the basis for their respective opinions and would each be cross examined about them, to place the jury in a position to evaluate their testimony in the context of the other evidence in the case. It is impossible to predict what the outcome of such a trial would be given the number of variables but it can be seen that it would have been fairer to all parties, including the experts who are part of such a divided community.

[15] If there had been evidence that Jade had previously suffered from sexsomnia the position would be different but, in the absence of such evidence, such questions would amount to a 'fishing expedition'.

[16] I.e. the jury would be entitled to conclude that the reason the defendant did not give evidence was that he had no answer to give, or none that would stand up to cross examination.

[17] If the jury are satisfied that there was a case for the defendant to answer at the time of his interview and that there was good reason for him to remain silent, they are entitled to conclude that the reason he did not answer questions was that he had no answer to give, or none that would stand up to investigation.

## 4 Conclusion

Ultimately Jade challenged the decision by the CPS to drop her case and, following a review they agreed that the case should not have been stopped and apologised unreservedly, but explained that they were unable to re-open the case as the suspect had been formally acquitted prior to the trial taking place. The CPS have since changed their guidance, stating that the Director of Legal Services needs to be notified whenever a prosecutor proposes not to charge or to stop a case arising from a defence of non-insane automatism (including sexsomnia). While clearly an additional level of oversight is welcome, we are still of the opinion that the threshold for diagnosis of parasomnia provided by forensic sleep medicine is far too low, meaning that often its mobilisation in a trial shifts the nature of the question at stake to whether there is sufficient history of parasomnias to conclude that a person was sleepwalking at the time, rather than focusing on whether sexual intercourse was non-consensual. While the location of the burden and standard of proof may enable undeserving claims of sexsomnia to be made, compliance by experts with the relevant rules and stringent application by the courts of the tests for admitting expert evidence should go some way towards mitigating the risk that they will succeed.

**Funding** The authors do not have any funding or competing interests to declare.

## References

American Academy of Sleep Medicine. 2014. *International Classification of Sleep Disorders*, 3rd ed. Darien: AASM Foundation.

American Law Institute. 1985. *Model Penal Code: Official Draft and Explanatory Notes: Complete Text of Model Penal Code as Adopted at the 1962 Annual Meeting of the American Law Institute at Washington, D.C., May 24, 1962.* Philadelphia, PA: The Institute.

American Psychiatric Association. 2013. *Diagnostic and Statistical Manual of Mental Disorders*, 5th ed. Washington DC: APA.

*Bratty v A-G for Northern Ireland*. 1963. A.C. 386, HL.

Child, John, Hans Crombag, and Robert Sullivan. 2020. Defending the delusional, the irrational, and the dangerous. *Criminal Law Review* 4: 306–324.

Criminal Justice and Public Order Act. 1994. c.33.

Criminal Procedure (Insanity) Act. 1964. c.84.

Criminal Procedure Rules. 2020. SI 2020/759. https://www.legislation.gov.uk/uksi/2020/759/contents/made. Accessed 28 May 2024.

Criminal Practice Directions. 2023. https://www.judiciary.uk/wp-content/uploads/2023/04/Criminal-Practice-Directions-2023.pdf. Accessed 28 May 2024.

Crown Prosecution Service. 2021. Chapter 4: Tackling Rape Myths and Stereotypes. In *Legal Guidance. Rape and Sexual Offences*. Crown Prosecution Service. https://www.cps.gov.uk/legal-guidance/rape-and-sexual-offences-overview-and-index-2021-updated-guidance.

Davies, Gemma, and Emma Piasecki. 2016. No More Laissez Faire? Expert Evidence, Rule Changes and Reliability: Can More Effective Training for the Bar and Judiciary Prevent Miscarriages of Justice? *The Journal of Criminal Law* 80: 327–343.

Director of Public Prosecutions. 2018. *Code for Crown Prosecutors*. https://www.cps.gov.uk/publication/code-crown-prosecutors

Director of Public Prosecutions. 2020. *Rape and Serious Sexual Offences Strategy*. https://www.cps.gov.uk/sites/default/files/documents/publications/RASSO-2025-strategy.pdf

*DPP v Majewski*. 1977. A.C. 443, HL.

Ebrahim, Irshaad Osman. 2006. Somnambulistic Sexual Behaviour (Sexsomnia). *Journal of Clinical Forensic Medicine* 13: 219–224.

Ebrahim, Irshaad Osman, and Peter B. Fenwick. 2007. Response to Pressman 'Factors that Predispose, Prime and Precipitate NREM Parasomnias in Adults: Clinical and forensic implications.' *Sleep Medicine Reviews* 11: 241–243.

Ebrahim, Irshaad Osman, Peter B. Fenwick, Richard Marks, and Kevin W Peacock. 2005. Violence, Sleepwalking and the Criminal Law: Part 1: The Medical Aspects. *Criminal Law Review*, 601–613.

Eigen, Joel Peter. 2003. *Unconscious Crimes: Mental Absence and Criminal Responsibility in Victorian London*. Baltimore: Johns Hopkins University Press.

Gaudreau, Hannah, Steve Joncas, Antonio Zadra, and Jacques Montplaisir. 2000. Dynamics of Slow Wave Activity During the NREM Sleep of Sleepwalkers and Control Subjects. *Sleep* 23: 1–6.

Idzikowski, Chris. 2014. An Essay on Sleep-Related Sexual Behaviours and Offences Related to Sexual Behaviours. In *Sleep and its Disorders Affect Society*, ed. Chris Idzikowski, 51–76. https://www.intechopen.com/chapters/47467. Accessed 28 May 2024.

Jackson, Adam, Gethin Rees, and Natalie Wortley. 2015. Sleep Disorders/Sexsomnia: The Role of the Expert and the External/Internal Factor Dichotomy. In *Mental Condition Defences and the Criminal Justice System: Perspectives From Law and Medicine*, ed. Ben Livings, Alan Reed, and Natalie Wake, 236–274. Cambridge: Cambridge Scholars Publishing.

Law Commission, *Criminal Liability: Insanity and Automatism. A Discussion Paper.* 2013. https://cloud-platform-e218f50a4812967ba1215eaecede923f.s3.amazonaws.com/uploads/sites/30/2015/06/insanity_discussion.pdf. Accessed 18 September 2024.

*M'Naghten's Case.* 1843. 4 St Tr NS 847, HL.

Mangan, Michael. 2001. *Sleepsex: Uncovered.* Bloomington, IN: Xlibris.corp

Melechi, Antonio. 2003. *Fugitive Minds: On Madness, Sleep and Other Twilight Afflictions.* London: William Heinemann Ltd.

Mental Heath Act. 1983. c.20.

Ministry of Justice, *Achieving Best Evidence in Criminal Proceedings: Guidance on Interviewing Victims and Witnesses, and Guidance on Using Special Measures.* 2022. https://assets.publishing.service.gov.uk/media/6492e26c103ca6001303a331/achieving-best-evidence-criminal-proceedings-2023.pdf. Accessed 18 September 2024.

PA Media. 2019. Man Was Sleeping When He Sexually Assaulted Woman, Jury Finds. The Guardian, August 20.

*Parks v R.* 1992. 2 S.C.R. 871

Pressman, Mark. 2007. Factors That Predispose, Prime and Precipitate NREM Parasomnias in Adults: Clinical and Forensic Implications. *Sleep Medicine Reviews* 11: 5–30.

Pressman, Mark. 2013. Sleepwalking, Amnesia, Comorbid Conditions and Triggers: Effects of Recall and Other Methodological Biases. *Sleep* 36: 1757–1758.

Pressman, Mark, Carlos Schenck, Mark Mahowald, and Michel Cramer Bornemann. 2007a. Sleep Science in the Courtroom. *Journal of Forensic and Legal Medicine.* 14: 108–111.

Pressman, Mark, Mark Mahowald, Carlos Schenck, and Michel Cramer Bornemann. 2007b. Alcohol-Induced Sleepwalking or Confusional Arousal as a Defense to Criminal Behavior: A Review of the Scientific Evidence and Forensic Considerations. *Journal of Sleep Research* 16: 198–212.

*R v Bilton* (unreported) *The Guardian.* 2005.

*R v Burgess.* 1991. 2 Q.B. 92, CA (Crim Div)

*R v C.* 2013. EWCA Crim 223.

R v Davies (unreported) *The Times.* 2006.

*R v Dlugosz.* 2013. EWCA Crim 2.

*R v Heard.* 2007. EWCA Crim 125.

*R v Hennessy.* 1989. 1 W.L.R. 287, CA (Crim Div).

*R v Jaco*bs. 2023. EWCA Crim 1503.

*R v Kemp.* 1957. 1 Q.B. 399, Assizes.

*R v Quick.* 1973. Q.B. 910, CA (Crim Div).

*R v Sheehan & Moore.* 1975. 1 W.L.R. 739, CA.

*R v Silverlock.* 1894. 2 Q.B. 766, QBD.

*R v Stubbs.* 2006. EWCA Crim 2312.

*R v Sullivan*. 1984. A.C. 156, HL.
*R v Taj*. 2018. EWCA Crim 1743.
*R v Tolson*. 1889. 23 Q.B.D. 168, CCR.
*R v Turner*. 1975. Q.B. 834, CA (Crim Div).
Rabey v R. 1980. 2 S.C.R. 513.
Rees, Gethin, and Deborah White. 2022. Judging Post-Controversy Expertise: Judicial Discretion and Scientific Marginalisation in the Courtroom. *Science as Culture* 32: 109–131.
Sexual Offences Act. 2003. c.42.
Youth Justice and Criminal Evidence Act. 1999. c.23.

# Accounts of Non-resistance in Rape Verdicts: The Psychological Freeze Response Model and the State of Liminality

*Solveig Laugerud*

## 1 Introduction

Sexual violence can be considered an 'essentially contested concept' (Gallie 1955), with disagreements concerning the issues of force and physical resistance being particularly evident. Both common understandings and legal definitions of rape have changed considerably in recent decades, although disagreements concerning force and resistance seem to persist. In this context, resistance usually means physical resistance or verbal resistance in the sense of screaming for help, not necessarily attempts to talk oneself out of the situation or attempts to escape assault in more subtle ways (Ullman 2007). While the law in many jurisdictions now includes definitions that do not (solely) rely on force and resistance, instead emphasising consent or incapacity, police, legal actors, and other parties may still expect victims to resist (Chalmers et al. 2021; de Heer and Jones 2023; Houge and Laugerud 2023). This situation represents a serious cause for concern, given how victims tend to become silent and

S. Laugerud (✉)
University of Oslo, Oslo, Norway
e-mail: solveig.laugerud@jus.uio.no



R. E. Keyse et al. (eds.), *Sexual Violence in Medicine and Psychiatry*, Genders and Sexualities in History,
https://doi.org/10.1007/978-3-032-10800-5_8

apparently passive when facing sexual assault (Ullman 2007). The criminal justice system has accordingly been criticised for not taking seriously rapes in which the victims do not physically resist the assault (de Heer and Jones 2023; Schiewe 2019). Strong belief in the idea that 'real' rapes are violent and that 'real' victims attempt to fight off their attacker has been identified as the central reason why most rape cases are not prosecuted or fail to result in conviction (Chalmers et al. 2021; Conaghan and Russell 2014; Smith and Skinner 2017; Temkin et al. 2016). To overcome these apparently commonsensical ideas within the criminal justice system, it has been argued that the system needs to be augmented with expert knowledge of how people react to potentially traumatising incidents in terms of psychological evidence, expert testimony, jury education, and trauma-informed practices (Campbell 2022; de Heer and Jones 2023; Ellison 2018; Ellison and Munro 2017).

Psychological knowledge is in other words considered necessary in rape cases to explain seemingly counterintuitive victim behaviour. Indeed, the aim of submitting psychological evidence is to normalise reactions and behaviours on the part of victims that people believe to be abnormal following an assault. For example, it has been argued that it is normal to not report a potentially traumatising experience to the police immediately after the incident, that it is common for victims to take a shower after a rape rather than to immediately go to the hospital to undergo a forensic medical examination, and that it is not unusual to have only fragmented memories of the incident (Ellison and Munro 2017; Ellison 2005). More recently, it has also been argued that trauma may explain why many rape victims freeze or do not attempt to resist or fight off the attacker when assaulted (de Heer and Jones 2023). To freeze or experience tonic immobility suggests that a person is unable to act or speak due to experiencing intense fear. This phenomenon has been characterised as trauma-induced immobility or involuntary incapacitation, something that de Heer and Jones (2023) believe the criminal justice system should consider as evidence of non-consent during rape trials. Before the freeze response model was developed, other psychological concepts were considered. For instance, Bourke (2012) shows how forensic descriptions and accounts of rape during the nineteenth century alleged that the victim had become *insensible* during the attack. Here, insensibility did not refer to unconsciousness, but a state in which it was difficult to move the body, speak and reason, in part because of fear.

The freeze response model explains rape victims' apparently passive response to their assault with a scientific account that emphasises the aspect of fear. Accordingly, the framework fits well with both medical and legal understandings of rape. In Norway, unlike in some other countries, the freeze response is acknowledged by the criminal justice system as a possible and legitimate response to sexual violence (Houge and Laugerud 2023). However, it is not common for courts to consider the freeze response as evidence of non-consent, even though rape complainants increasingly report a freeze reaction after receiving information about this phenomenon via psychoeducation at the hospital and forensic medical experts testify to it during trials. In this chapter, I will analyse Norwegian case law to investigate the use of the freeze response model in rape verdicts delivered by appellate courts. My purpose is to examine how a scientific biomedical model of fear performs in criminal trials and to compare it with competing models that explain victims' apparent passive response to rape. These competing models include sleep, intoxication, and in-between positions conceptualised as liminal hotspots (Houge and Laugerud 2023; Laugerud 2023a, b; Stenner et al. 2017). Ultimately, my aim is to further conceptualise victims' responses to rape.

Conceptualising victims' apparent lack of resistance as part of a psychological trauma model entails the scientification of victims' responses to rape. Resorting to science tends to lend authority to statements and may strengthen victims' credibility due to legitimising behaviours that others deem irrational. Given that the judicial system is characterised by a range of expectations, the ability to account for one's apparently unseemly behaviour (e.g., lack of resistance during an assault) is crucial to achieving credibility. An account is a verbal device employed to bridge the gap between one's own action and others' expectations (Scott and Lyman 1968). A common expectation in court (and elsewhere) entails displaying the will to resist unwanted sexual acts. Thus, failure to do so must be accompanied by a convincing account that excuses or justifies behaviour that is generally perceived as untoward. This means that when victims evoke the freeze response model during their testimony in court, it serves to bridge the gap between their previous actions and the court's expectations of resistance when facing an assault. This chapter will critically examine the ways in which medical and legal knowledge in this regard co-constitute each other and how medical knowledge is applied in response to others' expectations.

## 2 Conceptualising Non-Resistance: The Freeze Response and Liminal Hotspots

To be scared stiff or frozen are common expressions that refer to an embodied response to fear. These expressions are increasingly appearing in institutional contexts dealing with sexual violence in a more scientific manner, such as with the freeze/flight/fight model that includes the condition of tonic immobility (paralysis). This model is based on a fear hypothesis suggesting that when non-human and human animals are faced with extreme fear and physical restraint (e.g., actual or perceived capture or entrapment), they may experience paralysis—that is, an inability to speak or act (Marx et al. 2008). According to Marx et al. (2008), the terms *freeze* and *tonic immobility* are commonly confused but actually represent different responses within the defence cascade. *Freeze* is the initial response whereby the animal ceases all movement to orient itself toward the potential threat and prepare for action, and it 'is associated with increased responsivity to stimuli, an alert posture and volitional action tendencies' (Marx et al. 2008, 75). *Tonic immobility* is the last response and occurs after an unsuccessful escape or attempt at resistance. It is associated with physical immobility and muscular rigidity, even though the body is in a highly alert state. Marx et al. (2008) argue that tonic immobility is relevant in sexual assault cases, given how such an assault is a form of trauma that entails both fear and entrapment. A few studies have investigated tonic immobility responses among rape victims. One study conducted in the United States shows that 65% of rape victims reported not physically resisting the attack while 38% reported not verbally resisting the attack (de Heer and Jones 2017), and in a Swedish study, 70% of rape victims reported involuntary immobility (Möller et al. 2017).

The freeze response model has been associated with psychological trauma. The shift to trauma-informed practices in various institutions has also prompted the development of psychoeducation—that is, an intervention that involves educating patients and translating knowledge regarding psychological trauma for them through dialogue (Torielli 2020). This knowledge includes common reactions to trauma, symptoms of post-traumatic stress disorder (PTSD), and coping skills. A basic aspect of psychoeducation involves informing the patient about the freeze, flight, and fight responses. The aim is to reduce any feelings of shame and strengthen the understanding of common and normal responses to traumatic experiences.

The freeze response model may explain the nature and meaning of fear in some rape cases. A study of mock jury deliberations shows how the freeze response has, to some degree at least, become part of such deliberations, although juries tend to draw a distinction between violent stranger rapes and acquaintance rapes (Chalmers et al. 2021). Mann (2023) reflects on the apparent paradox of applying the freeze response model to commonplace rape, arguing that the fear in this context is not the fear of death or extreme physical harm, but of what she refers to as 'social death.' She argues that social death in relation to non-violent rape entails immediate and strong feelings of shame, annihilation, and degradation. Mann (2023) questions the ways in which fear is conceptualised in commonplace rapes, although she does not question the fear hypothesis itself, which is what I intend to do in the forthcoming analysis.

My starting point is the fact that many commonplace rapes involve intoxication and/or sleep, which typically involves alterations in consciousness in which the complainant struggles to make sense of what is happening and, therefore, is unable to resist the sexual acts (Laugerud 2023a, b). Alcohol-related rapes may be characterised by a social interaction shaped by high levels of intoxication, which may lead to a chaotic, confusing, or ambivalent experience. Here, the individual may become entangled and ultimately trapped in a destructive flow of events, which rob victims of self-control and agency that leaves them confused and harmed (Tutenges et al. 2019). By contrast, sleep-related rapes typically begin when the victim is asleep and proceed through the transition from the state of sleep to the state of wakefulness (Laugerud 2023a, b). Both types of rapes involve a situation in which victims move between various levels of reduced consciousness wherein they are neither completely unconscious nor completely awake, although they lack an embodied ability to act (Heyes 2015; Laugerud 2023a, b; Williams 2005; Williams and Crossley 2008).

The transitional state between sleep and wakefulness can be characterised as a liminal state in which a person experiences lethargy in the limbs and a loosening of their associative processes (Schwenger 2012; Williams and Crossley 2008). Additionally, this transitional state has been described as recessive and entailing sensitivity to outer stimuli (Leder 1990). This double meaning creates a sense of ambiguity that complicates the interpretation of liminal states. Liminality, according to Stenner

(2021, 3), 'involves a temporary suspension of limits that permits a transition to a new set of limits.' In this sense, it can be characterised as involving 'processes of becoming.' Liminality can also be described as each of "both/and" and 'neither/nor,' as being both awake and asleep simultaneously implies being neither awake nor asleep.

Moreover, I suggest that the transitional states between sleep and wakefulness, when disturbed by a sexual violation, can be perceived as liminal hotspots. Here, a liminal hotspot is 'an occasion of sustained uncertainty, ambivalence and tension in which people feel "caught suspended" in the limbo of an in-between phase of transition' (Stenner et al. 2017, 141–142). Thus, it is a happening, a sort of interruption of something else, that becomes permanent, leaving the people involved feeling trapped in enduring liminality. The dynamics of liminal hotspots are paradox, paralysis, and polarisation.

## 3 Methodology

In this chapter, I analyse Norwegian case law to investigate the use of the freeze response model in legal decisions regarding rape. I have selected all the rape verdicts delivered by Norwegian appellate courts that include a reference to the freeze response. I examine when and how this model becomes relevant in relation to rape verdicts and unpack the ways in which it matters (or not) in terms of the processing of rape cases. I also compare verdicts concerning incapacitated rape with verdicts concerning coerced rape to determine the appropriateness of a model of fear when it comes to explaining non-consent. The purpose of this chapter is to consider how a scientific biomedical model of fear performs in legal processes and to compare it with competing models that explain rape victims' apparent passive response. The aim is to further conceptualise victims' responses to rape.

For the analysis, I select data from the 'Lovdata' database, which includes all the verdicts delivered by appellate courts. I search for all the decisions made concerning the Norwegian rape provision (LOV-2005-05-20-28-§291) that include at least one of the following search terms: 'freeze' in both Norwegian ('frys' and 'frøs or frøys,' which refer to the past tense) and English (it is also common to use the English word in Norway), 'paralyzed' ('lammelse' or 'lamslått' in Norwegian), 'become stiff' ('stivne'[1] in Norwegian), and tonic immobility ('tonisk immobilitet' in Norwegian). All the search words are truncated and include synonyms in the database. The search results in 41 decisions dating back to 2018. I manually sort through the decisions to check whether they are relevant and exclude cases concerning incestuous relations or victims under the age of 16. Several decisions are not relevant due to 'freeze' being used as an expression concerning being cold or the like. Thus, my final sample comprises 28 decisions. The selected cases involve decisions made on the basis of §291a and b (Penal Code 2005), which state the following:

> A penalty of imprisonment for a term not exceeding 10 years shall be applied to any person who **a.** obtains sexual activity through violence or threatening conduct, or **b.** engages in sexual activity with a person who is unconscious or for other reasons incapable of resisting the act.

The Norwegian legal system has few rules of evidence and none concerning expert evidence, except the prohibition of using a polygraph. In Norwegian criminal cases, appellate court decisions are made by a panel of judges (two professional and five lay judges) who deliberate together and reach a verdict. To convict, five votes are required. This means that if three of the seven judges vote for acquittal, the minority vote is decisive. It is fairly common to have dissenting decisions in rape trials. All the decisions need to be explained, reasoned, and justified. Written verdicts are typically three to five pages long if they include only one rape charge, or longer if they include more than one charge. Dissenting decisions need to include explanations of both points of view. Accordingly, the written documents include a summary of the case and the evidence, as well as an account of how the court reached its decision. Such accounts constitute the texts I analyse in this chapter. A written verdict does not represent an accurate summary of everything that occurred during the trial. Only aspects the judges consider important in relation to their decision are included. This suggests that the freeze response model might have been invoked in more cases, albeit without being mentioned in the written verdicts. This means that the present analysis is limited to what is included in the verdicts.

[1] In Norwegian, the most common expression is 'stiv av skrekk,' which is similar to the expression 'to be scared stiff.'

I perform a document analysis, focusing on what Asdal and Reinertsen (2022) refer to as 'issues.' The idea here is to follow an issue from its appearance through its transformations by tracing how, when, and where it appears through to the ways in which it transforms a legal case or is transformed by the case. An issue is not a neutral concept, such as the term 'case,' but rather a concept that provokes controversy (Asdal and Reinertsen 2022). An issue suggests something unsettled, something that needs to be decided on, where something is at stake. Therefore, it is important to consider what is at stake and for whom when examining the text. Moreover, focusing on issues allows for the investigation of problems and problematisations, because this is how disagreements tend to be framed. To identify the problem constructions in the texts, I question the assumptions taken for granted in the documents by tracing any claims that apparently do not require an explanation or justification and, therefore, are silenced in the texts. When issues are taken to court, they may be transformed, and legal transformations entail modifying work. The courts may modify an issue by turning a controversy into an everyday affair or vice versa. Modifying work may turn an issue around by redefining, reframing, retiming, or relocating it (Asdal 2015).

## 4 Analysis of the Freeze Response in Written Verdicts

In the data, the freeze response appears most often in incapacitated rapes (16 cases) and less often in forced rapes (11 cases). One case is counted in both categories due to including two different charges of rape in which the freeze response is relevant. The incapacity rapes resulted in ten convictions (in which four were dissenting decisions) and six acquittals (in which two were dissenting decisions), while the forced rapes resulted in nine convictions (in which one was a dissenting decision) and two acquittals.

The freeze response seems to be introduced by three different actors—namely, the complainant during their testimony after receiving psychoeducation at the hospital, a medical or psychological expert in terms of a statement (written report or oral testimony), and/or the prosecutor or court. When the freeze response is introduced, two transformations may occur. First, the freeze response may become a scientific explanation for a lack of physical resistance that is intended to prove the complainant to have been incapacitated. Here, expert knowledge may transform the case from a possible rape to a proven rape by serving as evidence. Second, the freeze response may simply become an account that attempts to bridge the gap between the complainant's previous actions (or lack thereof) and the court's expectations of resistance when facing an assault. In this regard, the case is not necessarily transformed, as the account itself does not prove incapacity or the case might end in an acquittal. Instead, the freeze response model itself may be transformed in terms of gaining a new meaning, and eventually, the understanding of sexual violence may also be transformed.

These transformations represent two continuous movements in the data that may sometimes overlap. The idea is not to categorise the cases as such; rather, it is to highlight two different forces at play within the data.

### *4.1 Case Transformations: the Freeze Response as Expert Evidence*

I consider the freeze response to be a form of expert knowledge in the analysis when it is introduced and/or explained by a medical or psychological expert and/or the complainant meets the model's criteria (experiencing strong fear and/or being or feeling trapped) and this is documented with evidence in court[2] Among the selected cases, one may be regarded as an exemplary case due to fulfilling all the criteria. In this case, a woman was sitting on a bench at a bus stop, waiting for the bus in the middle of the night after visiting a bar. She had been drinking and she was wearing headphones to listen to a podcast. A stranger sat down next to her and suddenly started to touch her back under her clothes. Then, he started touching her breast, and later, her genitals, all inside her clothes. According to the verdict, the complainant described the incident in the following way:

> The complainant has explained that she was unable to move during the incident and that she tried to shout "stop" and "help me," but there was no sound. She cried silently. She was able to move her eyes but could not make eye contact with people close by. (LB-2019-178835)

[2] It is important to emphasise that Norway does not have a corroboration rule. In fact, the Supreme court has stated that the courts are allowed to solely conduct a credibility assessment in cases of sexual assault.

Subsequently, the complainant managed to make eye contact with nearby witnesses, who helped her and testified to doing so in court. The court described their testimonies in this way:

> Witness C has explained that he saw the complainant crying when he became aware of the situation. She must have been crying for a while as her mascara had run down her face and partially solidified. She formed her mouth into a "help me," but he could not hear her voice. It was obvious to him that she needed help. Witness D has explained the same thing. When they managed to get the defendant away from the complainant, she was shaking. Her teeth chattered and she appeared to be in shock.

A medical expert who testified in court and also wrote an expert statement explained that the freeze response is an involuntary response to experienced danger in which the body becomes paralyzed and the voice may disappear. Additionally, the body may become cold and start to shake. The expert further emphasised that it is common to freeze during a rape. Based on the eyewitnesses' accounts and the expert's statement, the court stated that it is convinced beyond reasonable doubt that the complainant had a freeze response due to strong fear and, therefore, could not resist the sexual assault. In this case, the complainant fulfilled the criteria of the freeze response model (e.g., experiencing strong fear, paralysis, lack of voice, and tremors), and most importantly, this fact was documented by an expert witness *and* eyewitnesses. The case clearly shows how the freeze response model may become a scientific explanation for a complainant's lack of resistance. The model performs well here, as the incident took place in public, in a context that is not normally associated with sex, and where people witnessed it. In other words, the freeze response model transformed the case by proving the complainant to have been incapacitated and raped. As an exemplary case, it functions as a norm for how similar cases should be deliberated and decided on.

Still, few cases perform in the same manner as the case above. Most cases under this heading include a description of the fear the complainant felt and an expert statement, but eyewitness statements are rare, as in most kinds of rape cases. However, in one case that resulted in an acquittal (LF-2020-1855), a witness over*heard* the alleged rape that occurred in a public toilet. The witness was in the cubicle next to the cubicle where the incident took place. The witness overheard noises that she interpreted as sex, which the court described as follows.

> The witness did not have the impression that anything involuntary was happening in the neighbouring cubicle. She explained that it seemed to be consensual and that nothing indicated otherwise.

Later, another witness (the complainant's sister) entered the toilet block and heard the same noises and some mumbling. When she heard her sister say 'no, no, not there, not there,' she became worried and went to seek help. The complainant explained that she had tried to resist the sexual acts, but had eventually given up, before freezing. The two witnesses overheard rather than observed the incident in question. As the first witness stated she did not hear anything unusual with regard to the sexual encounter, her testimony undermined rather than substantiated the rape claim. This is perhaps unsurprising considering how a freeze response may be perceived as a muted response. It is not possible to hear a body stiffen or a lack of voice. However, it is possible to hear some forms of resistance, and it is possible that the lack of sounds indicating resistance was interpreted as consent or, at least, that it contradicted the complainant's claim that she resisted before she gave up. These cases suggest that the *freeze* response needs to be documented, not only by an expert witness but through an eyewitness account. This means that an eyewitness account is more valued than an expert account. Although witnesses always interpret what they see, a freeze response has more visual than audial features and so needs to be observed rather than overheard. This also means that other visual representations, such as video recordings, may be able to document a freeze reaction.

In some cases, the alleged rape was recorded by surveillance cameras or smartphones. This occurred in case LB-2020-156732, in which the defendant was accused of sexually assaulting several women on various occasions. One incident occurred in a bar, when the accused had sat down with a group of women he did not know. This is how the court described the incident based on the video recording:

> The video shows that the defendant took every opportunity to touch the complainant while they were sitting next to each other, for example, by leaning over her and placing his hand on her arm while laughing, and by grabbing her hand for a high five. On some occasions, he also touched her thigh. Based on the video and the testimony before the Court of Appeal, the sexual act in question occurred when the defendant grabbed the complainant's arm and pulled her forward so that he could reach behind her hip with his hand. He then put his hand inside her panties,

> where he touched her anal opening with his fingers. After pulling his hand back up, he smelled and licked his fingers right in front of her face. This happened several times at short intervals. The complainant sat rather stiffly on the sofa before she stood up abruptly and went home.

The complainant explained that the incident occurred out of the blue and, therefore, caught her by surprise. For this reason, she had no opportunity to react. Moreover, she was so shocked that she froze and was unable to resist the defendant's continuous acts. The video recording allowed the court to see for themselves the defendant's acts and the complainant's stiff posture. Visual evidence is persuasive because it tends to be perceived as a substitute for seeing the *real* thing—that is, as an unmediated representation of the world (Mnookin 1998). For this reason, the evidentiary capacity of photographic evidence may gain uncritical trust (Ehrlich 2019). It may also provide common perceptual and conceptual ground between the judges, the complainant, and the expert, something that may strengthen their belief in having arrived at the correct decision (Feigenson 2014). Documentation such as eyewitnesses' accounts and visual evidence suggests that it is the observable feature of the freeze model that counts when proving the complainant could not resist the assault. This indicates two things. First, incidents that take place in public settings are more likely to be documented, as the previous examples illustrate. Second, medical models must rely on measurable features to perform well in legal settings. The measurable features of the freeze response model include 'motor inhibition, tremors, eye closure, increased respiration, and reduced core body temperature, or a subjective feeling of coldness' (Marx et al. 2008, 80). The two cases described above that ended in a conviction include some of these features. The reliance on measurable features shows how complex human behaviour is reduced to simple biological explanations. When the law relies on the freeze response model in this manner, it participates in the medicalisation of behaviour generally deemed incomprehensible or problematic (Nelkin and Tancredi 1989).

Most of the cases were not visually documented but included expert statements and fulfilled the model's criteria. One important feature of the freeze response model is the fact that it is based on a hypothesis of fear. This means that fear must be present in a case to render the claim of a freeze reaction credible. In some cases, fear is evident. In case LB-2022-155047, a woman who was heavily intoxicated after a night out was attacked by a stranger on her way home. The attack happened after she fell down a steep slope and lost her phone. She was searching for her phone in the bushes when one of the accused appeared. She was pushed to the ground and raped. She was unable to resist and completely froze. She stated that she thought she was going to be killed. Shortly afterwards, the accused and his friend drove her to their apartment where they both raped her on the kitchen floor. She said she did not resist it, although she did say 'no.' She explained that she was scared stiff because she thought she was going to be killed. An expert witness explained the freeze response to the court, which stated the following:

> The Court of Appeal is convinced that the victim experienced a so-called freeze reaction due to her high level of intoxication and strong fear. The expert witness described this as one of three main responses to experienced danger. The other two are flight and fight. [The expert] explained that the brain makes a quick decision regarding which of these reactions ensures the best chance of survival and chooses that one. The complainant was intoxicated, in a vulnerable situation after falling down the steep slope, and was facing two strange men—she feared for her life.

Regarding the second incident, the court stated:

> She was in a strange apartment, on the floor, without her cell phone, with two unknown men—and she thought she was going to die. Shortly before, she had been transported to the apartment via car by the unknown men—and she had been assaulted by one of them on a steep slope in the city.

The court highlighted how terrifying these incidents must have been for the complainant. The case contained numerous elements that both individually and collectively could be regarded as highly frightening. Multiple unknown perpetrators, abduction, and a series of rapes render the case rather extreme. Thus, it makes sense and is convincing that the complainant froze because she was so scared. Additionally, the court might have been convinced by the expert witness who relied on a neurobiological framing, which tend to give authority to statements. In other and more commonplace rape cases, the threatening features of the incidents may be more subtle, ambiguous, and/or contested.

A more commonplace rape is a rape that occurs in someone's home, among people who know each other, and without the use of physical force. An example in which an expert statement regarding the freeze reaction was included can be seen in case LB-2022-150937. Here, three friends (two women and one man) went to sleep in the same bed after a long Independence Day celebration. They had all been drinking quite a lot of alcohol. The women claimed that their male friend had started to grope them while they were trying to sleep. After a while, one of them got up and left the room. The other one fell asleep and woke up while being raped. She explained that she was unable to move or make a sound, referring to the experience using expressions such as 'everything froze,' being 'paralysed' and 'stuck,' and having a 'claustrophobic feeling.' The court was convinced that she experienced a freeze reaction and stated based on an expert statement:

> The Court of Appeal points out that a freeze reaction is a non-volitional, instinctive reaction to perceived danger. A person who experiences a freeze reaction cannot therefore choose to act "more rationally." Studies have shown that freeze reactions are not uncommon among rape victims. In the Court of Appeal's view, there are several circumstances in the course of events that contributed to making the situation frightening for the complainant and that, therefore, help to explain why she reacted as she did. First, the Court of Appeal refers to the fact that she was asleep and woke up to find a person lying behind her pulling down her pants and panties. This is in itself a clearly threatening situation, and the Court of Appeal considers it entirely natural that the complainant reacted with fear. In addition to the fact that she had just woken up in a threatening situation that made her feel afraid, the Court of Appeal points out that the complainant must have been tired and fatigued after the party, which had lasted almost all night. It is not surprising that she was unable to think clearly in such a situation.

Moreover, in this case, the court emphasised how threatening the incident must have been for the complainant. However, the way in which the judges reasoned regarding this matter suggests that they assumed it would not be intuitive to the reader and/or that it had been a contested issue during trial. They offered several arguments to explain why the situation was threatening and did not simply state that it was, as in the previous example. The court further underlined how threatening it must have been by using formulations such as 'clearly,' 'natural,' and 'not surprising' when explaining that the complainant had experienced fear in that situation. An incident that takes place at home, among friends, and without the use of physical force may appear less threatening and more ambiguous and so be more contested than incidents resembling a *violent stranger rape* and a *gang rape*, as in the earlier example. The ambiguity is connected to the different sources of fear. In the first example, it is connected to a threatening situation (outdoors, at night, multiple strangers, and abduction), while in the second example, it is connected to the complainant's condition (being exploited while asleep and intoxicated). A threatening situation is more readily available to document, which may make it easier to believe. *External threats*, as opposed to an *internal state* such as sleep, may also make more sense when perceived as frightening, given how sleep is commonly associated with both being in bed (the crime scene in this case) and engaging in consensual sex (sex being a bed-based activity initiated before and after sleep) (see Laugerud 2023a, b). External threats, as seen in the previous case involving abduction, may further resemble a *life-or-death scenario* in which the complainant fears for her life. This is the kind of fear that the freeze response model is built on. By contrast, waking up during a rape while lying in one's own bed may evoke a different kind of fear—that is a fear of annihilation and social death (Mann 2023). Even though the court concluded that the complainant must have experienced a freeze reaction after waking up while being raped, this matter was not decisive in terms of the court's decision to convict the defendant; rather, it added weight to the overall assessment of the other evidence in the case.

When fear is connected to sleep, sleep itself becomes the main issue and, therefore, must be proven. This is illustrated by a case that ended in an acquittal. This case included multiple charges of rape against several women, all on different occasions and while they were asleep at after-parties. In one instance, the complainant explained that she was asleep but was woken up by the assault and then instinctively froze. An expert testified in court to explain this condition and corroborate her claim. The court was not convinced that she was sleeping when the intercourse started, which shaped the court's perception of the complainant's lack of resistance:

> As accounted for above, the Court of Appeal does not find it proven that the complainant was still asleep when the sexual intercourse was initiated. The occurrence of an acute and paralysing freeze reaction is then cast in a completely different light than if the complainant were to wake up in the middle of the sexual intercourse.

In a situation without any clear signs of danger, it makes little sense to freeze unless the complainant was asleep, which the court considered unlikely. Accordingly, *fear* formed an essential aspect of the court's assessment. This is not surprising, given how the freeze response model is based on a hypothesis of strong fear (Marx et al. 2008). However, fear is primarily understood as arising from the danger associated with explicit threats of physical violence in a particular situation. Perceptions of fear are thus guided by common assumptions regarding violence and sexual violence in which (threats of) physical violence made in a public space by a stranger appear to be most readily and intuitively acknowledged as representative of proper danger. Only occasionally do the courts consider being taken by surprise and exploited due to an internal state of mind, such as sleep, to be a source of fear. Although fear is mentioned in some of the cases involving sleep and/or heavy intoxication (incapacitated rape) selected for the present analysis, it is simultaneously surprising how rare explicit descriptions of fear are in such cases. These rapes appear to be characterised by other characteristics, such as confusion, which I will demonstrate in the next section.

### *4.2 Transformation of the Model and Perceptions of Sexual Violence: The Freeze Response as an Account*

I consider the freeze response to be an account in the present analysis when the verdict includes a description of how the complainant referred to the term and/or similar terms but when it is not documented in any other ways, neither in terms of eyewitness observations nor expert statements.

The majority of cases that include a reference to the freeze response were prosecuted as incapacitated rapes due to the complainant being asleep and/or heavily intoxicated. These cases are more contested than forced rape cases in terms of more commonly ending in an acquittal and/or dissenting decision, and/or explicitly disputing the meaning of a lack of physical resistance. Similar to the last two cases discussed in the previous section, these cases typically involve a *woke-up-and-froze scenario* rather than a perceived *life-or-death scenario.* The analysis here, however, focuses on how the complainants' apparent passive response was explicitly disputed when not further documented and shows how the fear hypothesis does not necessarily fit the transitional state of waking up.

In a case (LH-2021-161475) in which colleagues had been partying together, two colleagues (the complainant and the accused) ended up heavily intoxicated at the complainant's apartment. After throwing up in the bathroom, the complainant went to bed to sleep. The accused went to bed in the living room. At some point, he moved into the bed where the complainant was sleeping. The complainant claimed that she woke up while being raped and froze. The case ended in a dissenting decision. The deciding minority acquitted the defendant due to being unconvinced that the complainant was incapacitated as a result of fear and sleep. This is how they argued their decision:

> The minority assumes that the complainant was asleep when the accused started touching her but that she was in a state of waking up before the sexual intercourse began. The minority cannot rule out that she was sufficiently awake to not be considered asleep. This is based on the fact that she registered that the accused touched her body in several places and that he held his hand over her genitals without touching them. She could also feel that he placed his penis between her thighs and then inserted it into her vagina. In its assessment, the minority has taken into account that the complainant thought she had gone to bed alone, that she did not know who was lying behind her in the bed, and that she was scared and confused.

Here, the deciding minority offered an argument against the complainant's claim that she was incapacitated and, therefore, unable to resist the assault. The minority focused on how to interpret the distinction between sleep and wakefulness, and they did not consider whether the complainant froze during the incident, something that the majority did consider, which I will return to below. The minority concluded that the complainant must have been wide awake because she was able to notice what was happening to her. This suggests that the minority did not recognise the notion that waking up constitutes a transition from one state to another in which it takes time and effort to become fully alert and ready to act. The transitional state between sleep and wakefulness has been described as a recessive state of being in which one is simultaneously sensitive to outer stimuli (Leder 1990). A transitional state may thus be characterised as an ambiguous state, as it includes elements of both states. This idea of being both absent (recessive) and present (sensitive) complicates interpretation of transitional states such as waking up (Laugerud 2023a, b). To be in-between sleep and wakefulness suggests a state of mind in which one is *both* asleep *and* awake while simultaneously being *neither* asleep *nor* awake (Stenner 2021). Even though the minority concluded that the complainant was awake and not asleep, it is clear that the question of how to interpret what constitutes sleep, legally speaking, was at the heart of the legal deliberations. The verdict included several references to the legal literature and case law concerning this issue, including the following:

> A person who is in a state of sleep whereby they are "distant" from themselves and therefore lack the ability to react to what is happening around them will be unable to resist the act [...]. The Court of Appeal assumes that it may nevertheless be the case that a person may be unable to resist sexual intercourse in the phase immediately after sleep, for example, where a person wakes up from a very heavy sleep but is unable to fully orientate themselves with regard to time, space, and whatever else is happening. To the extent that a person is in such a sleep-like state that the basic preconditions for action, such as conceptualization and physical disposition of the body are unattainable, this should be treated in the same way as sleep.

Here, the court described the phase of waking up as a process or transition characterised by disorientation, confusion, and uncertainty. The court further noted how alert wakefulness constitutes a precondition for action while sleep, as well as a sleep-like condition, restrain action. The ways in which the court described this transition or sleep-like condition resemble what Stenner (2021) referred to as a liminal state. This is a state in which a person has left one state (sleep) but not yet reached another (wakefulness). In other words, it is a process of becoming awake in which the limits of sleep temporary dissolve while the limits of wakefulness are still taking shape. The disruption of this transition by an assault may cause a feeling of being in limbo—that is, entrapped in enduring uncertainty, tension, and paralysis. Stenner et al. (2017) termed this a liminal hotspot.

The description of a sleep-like state that occurs during the transitional phase of waking up seems to resemble the confusion that the complainant in the most recent case example described, which was represented by the minority vote set out above. The minority still considered it a state of wakefulness, not a sleep-like condition, while the majority decided to avoid this question altogether:

> The majority assume that she was asleep when the accused started groping her, and that she was waking up before the intercourse was consummated.

> The majority also assume, as the minority have done, that the complainant thought that she had gone to bed alone, that she did not know who was behind her in bed, and that she was scared and confused. However, the majority find it proven beyond any reasonable doubt that she found this so frightening that she had a freeze reaction, as she has explained. She felt a "lump in her stomach" and could not move. She wanted to stop the action but could not do so. The physical disposition of her body was unattainable. Her reaction must also be viewed in the context of the fact that she had been in deep sleep and that she was affected by the night's alcohol consumption when the sexual intercourse took place. The majority do not find it necessary to consider whether the condition should be treated as a sleep-like condition, as the complainant's condition was in any case such that she was unable to resist the act.

The majority recognised the complainant's feelings and experience of paralysis, although they interpreted it as a freeze response rather than a sleep-like condition, even though the resemblance to the latter was clear. A sleep-like condition denotes an *internal sense of chaos* rather than an *external source of fear*. An internal and complex state of liminality with few observable features perhaps makes it easier to apply a simpler model of fear when establishing the facts of a case. The fluidity and ambiguity of liminality challenge fact-finding processes; however, when courts are asked to clarify the legal meaning of the process of waking up, they do address the complexity of liminality as a concept.

In a case (LB-2018-169937) that was appealed on grounds of both its facts and procedural issues, the court deliberated on the question of whether waking up in the middle of an assault satisfies part of the incapacity requirement of the rape provision—that is, 'unconscious or for other reasons incapable of resisting the act.' The court was divided into a majority and minority vote, with the minority vote consisting of (only) one lay judge.

> The fact that the victim woke up during the defendant's attempt and that he then continued his act until the victim managed to push him away, approximately one to two minutes after she woke up, does not indicate that the offence falls outside the scope of the provision. In the majority's view, it is irrelevant to the assessment of the criminal offense that the victim woke up while the attempted rape was in progress, whether the defendant then subjected the victim to violence or threats, and what resistance she

> showed at this time. When she woke up, the accused was already in the process of attempting to rape her.

The majority went on to explain why waking up satisfies part of the incapacity requirement:

> The decisive factor is whether the complainant is in a situation where she has no control over herself in relation to protecting her sexual autonomy. In the transition from sleep and in shock at what was going on, as well as while lying on her stomach with the defendant lying heavily on top of her, the victim was in a phase where, as she herself described it, she was prevented both physically and mentally from resisting the act, until she was able to react after a short time. The Court of Appeal is of the opinion that the phase immediately after sleep, in cases where the victim has not yet fully understood what is happening and has not regained physical control, can be equated with sleep and will in any event be covered by phrase "or for other reasons incapable of resisting."

This description of the liminal space of waking up suggests that waking up requires more than merely a sensibility to outer stimuli, as discussed earlier. To use the words of Williams and Crossley (2008), sleep constitutes a loss of an embodied grip on the world, a 'failure to be there fully in the body.' Waking up accordingly involves regaining an embodied grip and involvement in the situation to be able to understand what is going on and to act upon that understanding. This implies that resisting sexual acts entails an embodied response, not only an ability to either sense or move your body (Laugerud 2023b). In this case, however, the majority resorted to the freeze response model when stating the facts of the case—namely, that the complainant was asleep and confused about what to do when waking up. *Defining* incapacity appears to differ from *proving* it. Applying the freeze response model in addition to other models may also be an expression of how other models are not considered legitimate, not only that the logic of *fact finding* differs from the logic of *defining* a legal issue. The freeze response model has quickly been implemented in various institutional practices and also forms part of our common knowledge in the sense that we have everyday expressions that reflect the freeze reaction, such as 'being scared stiff.' For this reason, it may be tempting for legal decision-makers to add the freeze response model to other models in an effort to strengthen their argument.

## 5 Conclusion

The freeze response model is invoked in cases involving both forced rapes and incapacitated rapes, although most commonly in incapacitated rape cases. It is usually mentioned by the complainant after receiving psychoeducation, and it is also quite often explained by an expert statement. Occasionally it is documented by eyewitness statements or visual evidence, albeit typically only when the assault occurs in public. The present analysis shows that the freeze response model has the potential to serve as expert evidence that contributes to proving incapacity and/or rape under certain conditions. However, in most instances, the freeze response model does not seem to fit the conditions for two reasons. First, it does not seem to fit structurally. The freeze response model, as with biomedical models in general, is based on measurable features. As such, the model fits into the legal system well because of how the system relies upon documentation—that is, the process of making something visible in terms of evidence or eyewitness accounts. This means that the freeze response model may become relevant and serve as scientific evidence in cases that are possible to document. In rape cases, this usually means incidents that occur in public, when the perpetrator is a stranger, and where the use of force or violence is involved. In other words, in a very low number of cases. In most cases—that is, in commonplace rapes—it does not really fit. Second, it does not seem to fit semantically. The freeze response model relies on a hypothesis of strong fear, which is often associated with fear for one's life. It is imported from animal studies concerning *life-or-death* situations. Most rapes processed by the Norwegian legal system do not involve life-or-death scenarios or violence that invokes a similar type of fear. Instead, they are generally commonplace rapes that typically involve sleep and/or intoxication, with a common scenario being a *woke-up-and-froze* situation. Here, the *external source of fear* is less evident than the *internal sense of chaos* arising from the transition between various states of reduced consciousness. This implies that such cases typically concern *confusion* rather than *fear*. Thus, the challenge is to *document* rather than simply *define* this condition, a condition that is fluid, complex, and without obvious visual features to observe. Moreover, it is a condition that can be conceptualised as a liminal hotspot wherein a disruption of the transition from sleep to wakefulness may cause a feeling of entrapment accompanied by enduring uncertainty, tension, and paralysis. This model is more complex than the freeze response model and so requires sound investigation of testimonial evidence and reflected reasoning.

When the freeze response model is taken to court, it occasionally transforms the case. The present analysis shows that cases that fulfill the criteria of the freeze response model, that are explained by expert statements, and that are documented through eyewitness accounts or visual evidence succeed in proving a freeze response reaction and/or the rape itself. In such circumstances, the case is transformed from an alleged rape to a proven rape. However, this transformation is rare, given that most rape cases are difficult to document.

The present analysis also shows that in most cases, typically cases involving commonplace rapes, the freeze response model has only limited utility. In such cases, the complainant typically mentions freezing, although this phenomenon is not documented further and the model's criteria are not fulfilled. These cases typically concern a woke-up-and-froze scenario. Here, the cases are not transformed *because* of the freeze response model; rather, the freeze response model is transformed in the sense that it gains new meanings. In most cases that conclude with a freeze response, the model is not decisive in terms of the court's decision to convict the defendant, instead adding weight to the overall assessment of the other evidence in the case. This implies that woke-up-and-froze scenarios do result in convictions, mainly due to the existence of other compelling evidence. Accordingly, the courts contribute to the reconstruction of the freeze response as a general term for a lack of (physical) resistance, a term that has scientific legitimacy but lacks scientific content in its new version. Instead, it has become a popular-psychological concept (Gavey and Schmidt 2011). Indeed, the concept functions as an account, triggered by legal actors' questioning of resistance, that is intended to bridge the gap between the complainant's (lack of) actions and the legal actors' expectations of resistance (Scott and Lyman 1968). By utilising this concept, the complainant may avoid further scrutiny, as it carries weight and explains why they did not resist. This transformation also transforms conceptions of incapacitated rapes, as the freeze response associates them with an extremely fearsome situation such as a life-or-death situation. If the legal system instead acknowledged the liminality of waking up, there would be no need to apply the psychological freeze response model.

**Funding** This research is part of 'Evidently rape: Medical, legal and lay understandings of physical evidence in rape cases,' funded by UIO: Life Science, University of Oslo.

## References

Asdal, Kristin. 2015. What Is the Issue? The Transformative Capacity of Documents. *Distinktion: Journal of Social Theory* 16: 74–90. https://doi.org/10.1080/1600910X.2015.1022194.

Asdal, Kristin, and Hilde Reinertsen. 2022. *Doing Document Analysis : A Practice-Oriented Method*. London: SAGE.

Bourke, Joanna. 2012. Sexual Violence, Bodily Pain, and Trauma: A History. *Theory, Culture & Society* 29: 25–51. https://doi.org/10.1177/0263276412439406.

Campbell, Bradley A. 2022. Advancements in Trauma-Informed Training and Interviewing for Law Enforcement and Prosecutors. In *Sexual Assault Kits and Reforming the Response to Rape*, ed. Rachel E. Lovell and Jennifer Langhinrischsen-Rohling, 315–326. Abingdon: Routledge.

Chalmers, James, Fiona Leverick, and Vanessa Munro. 2021. The Provenance of What is Proven: Exploring (Mock) Jury Deliberation in Scottish Rape Trials. *Journal of Law and Society* 48: 226–249. https://doi.org/10.1111/jols.12287

Conaghan, Joanne, and Yvette Russell. 2014. Rape Myths, Law, and Feminist Research: 'Myths About Myths'? *Feminist Legal Studies* 22: 25–48. https://doi.org/10.1007/s10691-014-9259-z.

de Heer, Brook A., and Lynn C. Jones. 2017. Investigating the Self-Protective Potential of Immobility in Victims of Rape. *Violence and Victims* 2: 210–229. https://doi.org/10.1891/0886-6708.VV-D-15-00099.

de Heer, Brook A., and Lynn C. Jones. 2023. Tonic Immobility as a Defensive Trauma Response to Rape: Bridging Public Health and Law. *Violence against Women* 30: 3111–3139. https://doi.org/10.1177/10778012231174347.

Ehrlich, Susan. 2019. Well, I Saw the Picture': Semiotic Ideologies and the Unsettling of Normative Conceptions of Female Sexuality in the Steubenville Rape Trial. *Gender & Language* 13: 251–269.

Ellison, Louise. 2005. Closing the Credibility Gap: The Prosecutorial Use of Expert Witness Testimony in Sexual Assault Cases. *The International Journal of Evidence & Proof* 9: 239–268. https://doi.org/10.1350/ijep.2005.9.4.239.

Ellison, Louise. 2018. Credibility in Context: Jury Education and Intimate Partner Rape. *The International Journal of Evidence & Proof* 23: 263–281.

Ellison, Louise, and Vanessa Munro. 2017. Taking Trauma Seriously: Critical Reflections on the Criminal Justice Process. *The International Journal of Evidence & Proof* 21: 183–208. https://doi.org/10.1177/1365712716655168.

Feigenson, Neal. 2014. The Visual in Law: Some Problems for Legal Theory. *Law, Culture and the Humanities* 10: 13–23. https://doi.org/10.1177/1743872111421126.

Gallie, Walter Bryce. 1955. Essentially Contested Concepts. *Proceedings of the Aristotelian Society* 56: 167–198.

Gavey, Nicola, and Johanna Schmidt. 2011. 'Trauma of Rape' Discourse: A Double-Edged Template for Everyday Understandings of the Impact of Rape? *Violence against Women* 17: 433–456. https://doi.org/10.1177/1077801211404194.

Heyes, Cressida J. 2015. Dead to the World: Rape, Unconsciousness, and Social Media. *Signs: Journal of Women in Culture and Society* 41: 361–383. https://doi.org/10.1086/682964

Houge, Anette Bringedal, and Solveig Laugerud. 2023. 'Unconscious or for Other Reasons Incapable of Resisting': (Un)Protected Sexual Assault Under Norwegian Criminal Law. *Violence against Women*. https://doi.org/10.1177/10778012231181048.

Laugerud, Solveig. 2023a. Søvnens kraft: en analyse av begrepet og fenomenet sovevoldtekt. *Norsk sosiologisk tidsskrift* 7: 1–14. https://doi.org/10.18261/nost.7.2.1

Laugerud, Solveig. 2023b. The Victimised Body: Sexual Violence, Incapacity, and the Materialisation of Unconscious Bodies in Rape Verdicts. *Body & Society* 29: 29–52. https://doi.org/10.1177/1357034X231201942.

Leder, Drew. 1990. *The Absent Body*. Chicago, IL: University of Chicago Press.

Mann, Bonnie. 2023. Rape and Social Death. *Feminist Theory* 24: 377–397.

Marx, Brian P., John P. Forsyth, Gordon G. Gallup, and Tiffany Fusé. 2008. Tonic Immobility as an Evolved Predator Defense: Implications for Sexual Assault Survivors. *Clinical Psychology: Science and Practice* 15: 74–90.

Mnookin, Jennifer L. 1998. The Image of Truth: Photographic Evidence and the Power of Analogy. *Yale Journal of Law & the Humanities* 10: 1–74.

Möller, Anna, Hans Peter Söndergaard, and Lotti Helström. 2017. Tonic Immobility During Sexual Assault—A Common Reaction Predicting Post-Traumatic Stress Disorder and Severe Depression. *Acta Obstetricia et Gynecologica Scandinavica* 96: 932–938. https://doi.org/10.1111/aogs.13174

Nelkin, Dorothy, and Laurence R. Tancredi. 1989. *Dangerous Diagnostics : The Social Power of Biological Information*. New York: Basic Books.

Schiewe, Moriah. 2019. Tonic Immobility: The Fear-Freeze Response as a Forgotten Factor in Sexual Assault Laws. *DePaul Journal of Women Gender and the Law* 8: 1–28.

Schwenger, Peter. 2012. *At the Borders of Sleep: On Liminal Literature*. Minneapolis: University of Minnesota Press. https://doi.org/10.5749/minnesota/9780816679751.001.0001.

Scott, Marvin B., and Stanford M. Lyman. 1968. Accounts. *American Sociological Review* 33 (1): 46–62. https://doi.org/10.2307/2092239.

Smith, Olivia, and Tina Skinner. 2017. How Rape Myths Are Used and Challenged in Rape and Sexual Assault Trials. *Social & Legal Studies* 26: 441–466. https://doi.org/10.1177/0964663916680130.

Stenner, Paul. 2021. Theorising Liminality between Art and Life: The Liminal Sources of Cultural Experience. In *Experience on the Edge: Theorizing Liminality*, ed. by B. Wagoner and T. Zittoun, 3–42. Cham: Springer International Publishing. https://doi.org/10.1007/978-3-030-83171-4_1

Stenner, Paul, Monica Greco, and Johanna F. Motzkau. 2017. Introduction to the Special Issue on Liminal Hotspots. *Theory & Psychology* 27: 141–146. https://doi.org/10.1177/0959354316687867

Temkin, Jennifer, Jacqueline M. Gray, and Jastine Barrett. 2016. Different Functions of Rape Myth Use in Court: Findings From a Trial Observation Study. *Feminist Criminology* 13: 205–226. https://doi.org/10.1177/1557085116661627.

Torielli, Josie. 2020. Psychoeducation: Discussing Trauma with Patients. In *Sexual and Gender-Based Violence: A Complete Clinical Guide*, ed. by V. Ades, 19–36. Cham: Springer. https://doi.org/10.1007/978-3-030-38345-9

Tutenges, Sébastien., Sveinung Sandberg, and Willy Pedersen. 2019. Sexually Violent Effervescence: Understanding Sexual Assault Among Youth. *Sexualities* 23: 406–421. https://doi.org/10.1177/1363460719830342.

Ullman, Sarah E. 2007. A 10-Year Update of 'Review and Critique of Empirical Studies of Rape Avoidance.' *Criminal Justice and Behavior* 34: 411–429. https://doi.org/10.1177/0093854806297117.

Williams, Simon J. 2005. 'Liminal' Bodies?: Sleep, Death and Dying. In *Debating Biology*, ed. S. J. Williams, L. Birke, and G. A. Bendelow, 179–192. Abingdon: Routledge.

Williams, Simon J., and Nick Crossley. 2008. Introduction: Sleeping Bodies. *Body & Society* 14: 1–13. https://doi.org/10.1177/1357034X08096892.

# Historicising Medical and Psychiatric Responses to Sexual Violence

# 'Too Frightening and Inconceivable for a Balanced Mind': Sexual Violence and Mental Illness in Jewish Community Archives in Argentina

*Joanna Zofia Spyra*

## 1 Introduction

During my archival fieldwork in Buenos Aires in 2022, I found myself navigating the city's vibrant tapestry using the public transportation system, colloquially referred to as *colectivo* (bus transportation) or *subte* (subway). A conspicuous and recurrent observation during these journeys pertained to a municipal campaign poster bearing the slogan '*Ni Loca. Ni Perseguida. Ni Histérica. El Acoso Existe*' ('Not Crazy. Not Persecuted. Not Hysterical. Harassment Exists' [gendered female in Spanish]). This powerful message became a poignant part of my daily commute, sparking contemplation on the issue it tried to address. I later learned that the city had enacted a law aimed at preventing and penalising harassment in transportation and public spaces (Buenos Aires Government 2019). The campaign emphasises the significance of refraining from dismissing or stigmatising individuals grappling with experiences of sexual violence.

J. Z. Spyra (✉)
University of Bergen, Bergen, Norway
e-mail: joanna.spyra@uib.no





R. E. Keyse et al. (eds.), *Sexual Violence in Medicine and Psychiatry*, Genders and Sexualities in History,
https://doi.org/10.1007/978-3-032-10800-5_9

This advocacy struck a chord with me, as the issue of women's 'credibility' or the lack thereof emerged in the archival material I was analysing at the time.

In 1936, *Ezras Noshim* (Yiddish/Hebrew for 'the assistance of women', henceforth EN), a Jewish charity originally established to address concerns about the trafficking of women and girls in Argentina, documented cases of women considered to be mentally ill. Some of these women sought help from what EN described as 'imaginary enemies', presenting stories deemed 'too frightening and inconceivable for a balanced mind', leading the organisation to view women's claims with scepticism and disbelief. Noticing inconsistencies in the women's accounts, occasionally labelling them as 'unintelligible', EN consulted medical professionals who sometimes diagnosed the women with mental illness. Some of EN's charges focused their fears on certain individuals who were supposedly trying to push them into a 'promiscuous lifestyle'. EN noted that the medical assessment indicated that these 'persecutory delusions' and 'defects in their mental functions' were likely connected to 'sexual causes' and were rooted in 'failed romantic relationships' (Central Archives for the History of the Jewish People [henceforth CAHJP], AR/EN-3590, *Memoria de la 'Ezras Noshim' de Buenos Aires. Año 1936*, 53–56). Given EN's founding mission to combat prostitution and trafficking, women's fears of being forced into such a lifestyle may not have been surprising to the organisation. However, rather than validating these fears, some women were deemed mentally unwell. This brings attention to the differing ways in which certain women's fears were trivialised or pathologised, while others were viewed as legitimate and credible, suggesting inconsistencies in how EN recognised and responded to the vulnerability of those it aimed to protect. While it might be tempting to focus on narratives that emphasise the victimisation and oppression of the women involved, doing so would result in an oversimplification. EN's social workers navigated complex times marked by numerous and sometimes conflicting discourses regarding women's minds and bodies. Established in the early 1900s as an offshoot of the London-based Jewish Association for the Protection of Girls and Women (henceforth, JAPGW), EN originally focused on addressing concerns about the portrayal of Jews as key figures in the organised sex trade, with Argentina frequently identified as a major destination for such activities (Guy 1995; Schettini 2017). In collaboration with the League of Nations, JAPGW closely monitored sex trafficking, leading its South American branch to report cases (Knepper 2007). As EN's causes gained recognition within the wider Jewish community, the organisation achieved increased autonomy in 1926, gradually securing financial support and establishing an executive committee composed of 14 representatives from various local Jewish charities and societies. EN could intervene and advocate for Jewish women and minors in Argentine institutions such as police stations, hospitals, and immigration offices. Over time, its role expanded to assist Jewish women immigrants in various areas, such as resolving family and marital conflicts, facilitating medical care, addressing financial difficulties, and handling issues related to certificates of morality (Stadler 2020; Yarfitz 2013).

The chapter examines the records of EN from the early 1930s, providing specific examples from 1936, which marked the organisation's first explicit identification of cases related to 'mental illnesses'. These records reveal numerous facets potentially examinable as instances of sexual violence, although EN itself did not explicitly label them as such. The cases were mediated through EN, reflecting the cultural assumptions and perspectives of the organisation rather than those of the women themselves. Therefore, the chapter delves into not only the issue of sexual violence but also the communal responses to it, to answer the following questions: what difficulties are encountered when identifying sexual violence in historical sources? What might have been the underlying motivations driving EN's activities? How do historical narratives of sexual violence connect to contemporary accounts? In exploring these questions, the chapter contributes to broader methodological debates around archival approaches to historical research into sexual violence.

The chapter starts by delving into the methodological complexities of working with EN's archival collection, particularly in uncovering instances of sexual violence within its records. It introduces EN as a charitable organisation and seeks to place its role within a broader context, exploring how and why the charity may have addressed sexual violence, even when such issues were not always explicitly acknowledged as such. The discussion then moves to how EN facilitated medical care for the mentally ill and considers how both medical records and instances of sexual violence can be analysed through the lens of epistemic injustice. The chapter also addresses the challenges of applying terms like 'sexual violence' or 'sex work' to historical sources, noting how these concepts can both reveal and obscure past realities.[1] Moreover, it explores the link between historical and contemporary narratives, showing how simplified portrayals can help organisations secure funding and support for women while also simultaneously perpetuating misconceptions about sexual violence.

## 2 Methodological Approaches to Historical Sexual Violence in Community Archives

Methodological challenges in studying historical sexual violence, particularly the interpretation of incomplete and fragmented records, are a key focus of this chapter. The approach emphasises analysing material 'against the grain', requiring careful consideration of its potential, limitations, and biases while going beyond its surface-level content (Gordon 2018; Stoler 2009). Instead of relying on more 'traditional' sources like clinical cases from psychiatric hospitals, police reports, or court testimonies (Grey and Toledo 2022), the analysis focuses on voices interpreted by an organisation concerned with women's issues more broadly. The value of these records lies in their ability to capture cases of women who might not have directly interacted with institutions within the state apparatus and judicial systems. This use of community archives is significant and demonstrates how historians investigating sexual violence might seek out alternative archival collections, in order to access sources of information that may have been lost, not well preserved, or overlooked in other (state) contexts.

While the subject of Jewish women in early twentieth-century Argentina is frequently studied through the lens of gender, sexuality, and specifically sex work (Avni 2014; Deutsch 2010; Yarfitz 2019)—a topic that sparks polarised discussions within feminist discourses—the issue of historical sexual violence has rarely figured in these debates. This is striking because the award presented to contemporary organisations in Argentina committed to addressing violence against women bears the name of Raquel Liberman, a Polish Jewish sex worker whose testimonies played a pivotal role in the partial dismantling of a Jewish pimping organisation in Buenos Aires during the 1920s and 1930s (Derechos Humanos BA 2021). In Jewish historiography, sexual violence as an analytical category is frequently employed in the context of violence directed towards

[1] I want to note that I use the terms 'prostitute'/ 'prostitution' and 'sex worker'/ 'sex work' interchangeably, though I discuss the nuances of this terminology later in the text.

Jews by 'others'. A substantial body of literature has explored instances of sexual violence during the Holocaust, also delving into configurations beyond the 'conventional' male–female dynamic (Glowacka 2021; Hedgepeth and Saidel 2010; Person 2015). Through examining the records held within the *Ezras Noshim* archives, this chapter seeks to shift attention to what I term 'sexual violence from within', encompassing abuse inflicted by members of the community upon fellow members, including within the family or in other close interpersonal relationships. The term emphasises that this harm emanates from within the community (even when this community has its internal divisions), contrasting with external threats or violence. It also highlights internal responses to these issues, examining how they are managed within communal spaces.

In this chapter, I define sexual violence as a sexual act or behaviour that likely occurred without the full consent of the individuals involved. The definition acknowledges the challenge of applying current understandings of consent to historical contexts, recognising that the terminology may not perfectly align with past attitudes and language (Heberle 2014; Lammasniemi 2024). This encompasses behaviours that were potentially normalised by social, economic, or cultural pressures of the time, and might not have been legally recognised or prosecuted. It includes both explicit acts of aggression and more nuanced forms of coercion, such as emotional manipulation or economic dependency. I pay special attention to descriptions of distress related to potential sexual experiences, focusing on language that hints at emotional suffering and physical or psychological violence. The emphasis is on cases where evidence of enduring psychological harm points to experiences that undermined women's autonomy and dignity, while recognising that this perspective could be seen as problematic as some forms of mental illness may not stem from traumatic experiences (Bourke 2012). Simultaneously, the chapter critically explores the notion of agency, focusing on how power dynamics influence and shape individuals' capacity for autonomous actions. While some individuals whose stories appear in EN's records might have chosen to pursue prostitution voluntarily, their circumstances may have constrained their options. This is exemplified by the case of Raquel Liberman, mentioned earlier, whose precise motivations for entering prostitution remain unclear. Nonetheless, it is reasonable to infer that financial difficulties were a significant factor. Her situation—being widowed in a foreign country, and responsible for her children—created economic pressures that restricted her choices, thereby highlighting the complex interplay between personal agency and broader socio-economic forces.

## 3 Identifying Sexual Violence in *Ezras Noshim*'s Records

*EzrasNoshim's* archival collections are held at the Fundación IWO (*Instituto Judío de Investigación*/Institute for Jewish Research) archives in Buenos Aires, Argentina, and the Central Archives for the History of the Jewish People (CAHJP) in Jerusalem, Israel. Determining if the documents in Argentina are exact duplicates of those in Israel is difficult.[2] At the IWO archive, EN documents are divided into multiple boxes, without a catalogue or index. At the CAHJP, the EN catalogue points only to general themes. The sources in both locations are diverse, including correspondence, reports, photographs, newspaper clippings, statistics, and brochures. They are also multilingual: most are in Spanish, Yiddish, and Polish, with some correspondence in English, Russian, French, German, and Portuguese.[3] Many of the documents are in poor condition or are incomplete. At the IWO archive, researchers are not permitted to take photographs of the documents, whereas the CAHJP allow photography. Both archives require that records be anonymised; thus, the names of the women mentioned in this chapter have been altered.[4] While following these privacy guidelines is recommended, it may have unintended consequences. Anonymising historical records of sex workers and those considered mentally ill, especially those long deceased, could inadvertently reinforce the stigma associated with prostitution and mental illness (Hájková 2022, 197; Wright and Saucier 2012). However, when dealing with sexual violence cases, particularly those not explicitly labelled as such in historical records, it is essential to be acutely aware of the subjective nature of historical analysis when navigating these concerns.

[2] Efraim Zadoff, a historian, transported EN's documents from Argentina to Israel during the late 1970s Dirty War, following a request from AMIA's (Argentine Israelite Mutual Association) president to safeguard the collection in Jerusalem.

[3] All translations from Spanish are the author's own.

[4] The policies on anonymisation are not fixed. The ones discussed in this article were in effect from 2017 to 2022, based on the parameters of the author's research process rather than the specific timeframes of the policies themselves.

EN prepared reports for their own administrative purposes and to provide updates, for example to the JAPGW office in London. From 1930 to 1936, EN managed more than 5,500 cases—3,956 cases from 1930 to 1935, and 1589 in 1936—but only a select few were reported in detail, often chosen for their either exemplary or exceptional nature (CAHJP, AR/EN-3960, *Ezras Noshim. Obra Social de la Institución, Buenos Aires 1936*, 15; CAHJP, AR/EN-3590, *Memoria de la 'Ezras Noshim' de Buenos Aires. Año 1936*, 91). For instance, the 1936 report is written entirely in Spanish and includes about 90 pages detailing 18 individual cases selected by EN personnel. Besides the category of 'mentally ill women', EN classified cases into eight other groups: 'white slavery'; 'cases of disorderly behaviour in minors'; 'immigrant fiancés'; 'certificates of morality'; 'organisation of "*Jupe-Kadische*"' (religious marital ceremonies); '*get*' (Jewish divorce); 'marital conflicts' and 'miscellaneous' (CAHJP, AR/EN-3590, *Memoria de la 'Ezras Noshim' de Buenos Aires. Año 1936*, 2). Records from before 1936 show that EN was also actively engaged in protecting elderly women and managing cases of missing persons. Another significant issue was the predicament faced by women whose husbands had (usually deliberately) disappeared, leaving them without financial support and due to the Jewish religious laws, unable to remarry, trapping them in the state of 'marital limbo' as *agunot*.[5]

Many cases handled by EN dealt with overlapping concerns, underscoring the multifaceted nature of the issues EN sought to address. Each of these could encompass instances of sexual violence. For example, EN recorded the case of 18-year-old Dvora Shapiro, who was discovered abandoned and in poor health in a tenement in Buenos Aires. She had been living alone for several months, with rent paid by an unidentified stranger who never returned. Her relatives had disappeared, leaving her behind in the city. To address her health condition, EN placed her in the Jewish Hospital, where she initially remained calm. However, one night she woke up screaming and frightened, alleging an attempted rape by neighbouring patients. Upon examination she was diagnosed with 'a mental illness of sexual origin'. As the Jewish Hospital did not treat such conditions and her behaviour disrupted other patients, EN arranged her transfer to a mental institution in Córdoba province, with expenses

[5] The term *agunah* or *agunot* (plural) refers to women unable to secure a rabbinic divorce because of their husbands' unwillingness or inability. The literal meaning of this Hebrew word is 'chained' or 'anchored'.

covered by local Jewish Argentine charities. The report noted that Dvora's health did not improve (Ibid., 58–61).

The terms 'sexual origin' or 'sexual underpinning' used in Dvora's and other cases in EN's reports remain ambiguous and open to interpretation. It is unclear if these terms denote past sexual abuse, forced prostitution, or merely refer to Dvora's biological sex. The charity does not offer a clear definition of mental illness either. However, even in cases not specifically categorised as mental illness, EN employs highly medicalised language and places significant emphasis on assessing women's mental conditions. This approach reveals a complex attitude: on the one hand, it can be dismissive of women's experiences by questioning their mental stability and labelling their accounts as incoherent, yet on the other hand, it demonstrates a willingness to help by providing medical intervention and supporting their recovery.

Dvora was abandoned and without a support network, her condition was severe and visible, and reported to EN by others as she likely could not seek help herself due to her health. It is noteworthy that the term 'rape' rarely appears in EN's records and Dvora's fear of being raped speaks volumes about her possible past experiences. Her being found alone and exhibiting signs of distress at 18 suggests that the potential abuse likely took place when she was still a minor. The fact that EN secured a bed for her in a state hospital with funding from external institutions indicates the seriousness with which her condition was treated. It also demonstrates EN's authoritative role in assessing the mental state of Jewish women and determining the course of action to be taken on their behalf.

One could suggest tracking Dvora's medical records to learn about her subsequent whereabouts. That is, however, difficult due to the poor conditions of Argentine archives, which have been impacted by periods of political and economic instability.[6] This approach also raises potential privacy and ethical concerns. Jonathan Ablard notes that information on mentally ill patients in Argentina is scarce compared to the extensive data available in Western Europe and North America (Ablard 2008, 12). Early twentieth-century Argentine medical journals, such as *Archivos de Criminología, Medicina Legal y Psiquiatría* (Archives of Criminology, Legal

[6] Moreover, the 1994 terrorist bombing of the AMIA building in Buenos Aires destroyed valuable archival materials that were historically significant to Argentina's Jewish community.

Medicine, and Psychiatry), and *La Semana Médica* (Medical Weekly) often included anonymised case reports on mentally ill women but seldom mentioned their ethnicity (Dovio 2012). As a result, EN's records are among the few that explicitly document Jewish women patients and at least some aspects of their hospitalisation and treatment. Even if Dvora's records appear in a different archival setting, the anonymisation requirement makes it difficult for historians to determine or verify whether they are examining the same individual across various contexts.

Dvora's case underscores the methodological challenges inherent to studying historical sexual violence. The identification and definition of 'sexual violence' in archival records is complex: the term encompasses a broad spectrum of behaviours and relies heavily on subjective historical interpretation. Actions deemed sexual violence today might not have been recognised as such in the past. Similarly, understanding historical mental illness poses challenges. Rather than questioning past medical diagnoses and their causes, I aim to offer insights into how these experiences were perceived and categorised, and to explore the possible outcomes for those affected. If one accepts the premise that, for example, Dvora was indeed subjected to an act of sexual violence, the response to her situation can be analysed. The process began with observant bystanders who noticed her distress and informed EN about her condition. Subsequently, medical professionals identified the cause of her suffering and provided care. The organisation then committed to offering support, and continuously monitoring her well-being. Here, then, we see the importance of Dvora's connection to the Jewish community (whether this association was formal or informal, voluntary or involuntary), through which she was able to access care. Studying cases such as this one highlights the methodological benefits of researching in community archives, through which historians can find information about support mechanisms available to women at the time, outside the more 'traditional' sources associated with the criminal legal system.

## 4 Helping Women as a Jewish Communal Effort

*Ezras Noshim's* work took place in the context of a dramatically evolving social landscape. From the mid-1800s to the 1930s, Argentina attracted over six-and-a-half million migrants, ranking as the second most significant immigrant destination after the United States of America (Germani 1966, 166). The ruling elites actively promoted immigration to tackle low population density and advance the Republic's development. This endeavour was associated with a 'civilising mission', seeking to transform society based on a racial hierarchy of 'whiteness' and the creation of 'a healthy citizenry' (Rodriguez 2006, 4, 20–25, 33). However, the Nordic and Anglo-Saxon immigrants who were supposed to 'whiten' the population and contribute their 'superior traits' showed little interest in settling in Argentina (Rodriguez 2006, 5, 219; Bjerg 2016). The majority of immigrants came from Italy, followed by Spain, with a significant post-World War I influx from Poland (including Jews and non-Jews) forming the third largest group (Germani 1966, 167). This massive surge of newcomers transformed Argentina's social fabric, leading to strained medical infrastructure, a rapidly changing political climate, and growing hostility towards the absorption of new and 'less desirable' immigrants, particularly as right-wing sentiments grew in the 1930s (Reggiani 2010). Given the prevailing conditions, which also included the ambiguous racial classification of Jews and long-standing presumptions associating Jews with a perceived risk to public health, it became imperative to uplift the image of Jewish immigrants (Armus 2019; Granick 2021, 164–166; Lesser 1995, 7–8). It was necessary to provide an alternative narrative that could debunk detrimental stereotypes, countering notions of the Jewish community's alleged associations with disease or engagement in deviant sexual behaviour.

Although EN's objectives were not explicitly centred on health, the influence of the extensive medical surveillance implemented by the Argentine state can be seen within the organisation's records, most notably through the use of highly medicalised language when describing women's cases. For instance, the organisation used vivid imagery to denounce mothers engaged in prostitution, stating that they desecrated their own surroundings by 'violating the sacred principles of family, planting the germ of evil within the womb of their relatives' (CAHJP, AR/EN-3590, *Memoria de la 'Ezras Noshim' de Buenos Aires. Año 1936*, 5).

Antisemitism and medical discourses were not the only factors influencing or motivating EN. The charity was part of an interconnected mosaic of philanthropic organisations that tried to advance ideas of active and engaged citizenship, although 'citizenship' in the sense of nationality, was not automatically or easily granted (Bryce and Sheinin 2017, 5). Jewish charitable efforts in Argentina were part of a broader pattern; given that the majority of Buenos Aires' population were immigrants or of immigrant background, active participation in community life and national development was a widespread expectation shared by many (Kałczewiak 2019, 164). Immigrants, including Jews, were commonly engaged in various philanthropic activities as a way to integrate into society, contribute to local development, and address the needs of their communities (Bryce 2015). This involvement was not only a means of supporting those in need but also a way to forge connections with the larger society and align with the collective experiences of other immigrant groups in the city (Bryce and Sheinin 2017, 40–41). Emulating philanthropic practices could have facilitated greater integration for Jews. EN's support for Jewish women reflected ethnic pride, and in 1930, Helena R. de Aslán's appointment as the first female leader of EN underscored Jewish bourgeois women's dedication to charity and social advancement (Deutsch 2010, 223–226; Guy 2009). It is important to note that Jews in Argentina were not a monolithic entity, and many did not affiliate with community institutions. Some scholars argue that the reliance on community-based data in studies of Argentine Jewish history is excessive, as many research works, including this one, primarily draw from institutional records (Lesser and Rein 2008, 31–32). However, the women who came to EN's attention were not always included in its records by choice, nor were they necessarily connected to any other Jewish communal organisation.

## 5 Navigating Care: Hospitalisation, Epistemic Injustice, and Systematic Responses

In its 1936 annual report, *Ezras Noshim* noted an increase in cases of mental illness among the women it assisted and began categorising them as 'mentally ill women' for the first time. It is unclear why they chose to use this category more explicitly at that time, particularly since other cases from earlier periods could also have been classified as such. This shift may have been influenced by the recommendations of the League of Nations Advisory Committee on Traffic in Women and Children which in a 1936 report advocated for more psychological and psychiatric study of women, accessible psychiatric assistance, and better training for social workers (University of Southampton, Special Collection, MS 173, Archives of Jewish Care, 2/7, *The Jewish Association for the Protection of Girls, Women, and Children Report 1935–1936*, 36–38).

While not all EN cases involved (former) prostitutes, records from 1936 uncovered issues that echoed the concerns raised by the committee.

These included the necessity for hospitalisation for those diagnosed with mental illness, a heightened focus on protecting minors, and a perceived connection between women's intellectual capacities and promiscuity. For example, EN documented cases of married women displaying episodes of 'morbid jealousy' and physically aggressive behaviour towards their relatives. These were seen as indications of mental disturbances with sexual undertones, prompting the organisation to suggest 'systematic treatment' such as isolation and hospitalisation (CAHJP, AR/EN-3590, *Memoria de la 'Ezras Noshim' de Buenos Aires. Año 1936*, 54–55). However, some women who sought help from EN were deemed problematic and vexing, and such women were not offered medical intervention or evaluation. For instance, one young woman, Shoshana, suspected of having multiple sexual partners, was described as 'retarded' and her case was labelled as 'sexual pathology' (Ibid., 37). Another one, Judith, was noted for her 'awakened intelligence' and temperament after changing lovers twice in one year (Ibid., 38–40). These suggest that EN was particularly concerned with the moral and physical well-being of women, often conflating their mental abilities with their sexual behaviour, and reflecting broader societal anxieties about the role and conduct of women during that era.

Gaining admission for mentally ill individuals to state hospitals posed significant challenges due to severe overcrowding. For example, in 1934, *El Hospital Nacional de Alienadas* (National Hospital for Mentally Ill Women) in Buenos Aires, which had been designed to accommodate 1600 patients, provided care for more than 3000 individuals (Ablard 2009, 226). In 1936, EN reported that it managed to secure beds for five women with urgent and essential hospitalisation needs through what they called 'certain connections' (CAHJP, AR/EN-3590, *Memoria de la 'Ezras Noshim' de Buenos Aires. Año 1936*, 56), demonstrating the importance of the organisation for women accessing care.

Statistics from Argentine psychiatric hospitals indicated a rise in the number of immigrant patients, particularly from eastern Europe, during the interwar period (Ablard 2008, 85–86). A significant challenge accompanying this demographic shift was the communication between doctors and patients. Language barriers and cultural misunderstandings led to incorrect and significantly delayed diagnoses (Golcman 2017, 112). Beyond seeking medical opinions, the sources show that EN closely followed the hospitalisation of their charges. The relatively short hospital stays, typically lasting a few months for women with EN's support, imply quicker diagnoses and treatment compared to patients without such assistance. This suggests that EN not only facilitated referrals to appropriate institutions but also most likely served as an 'interpreter,' both in terms of language and cultural mediation.

In a medical context, the spoken account becomes a valuable source of information that aids in understanding the patient's health status, identifying potential causes of symptoms, and formulating an accurate diagnosis. This is similar to cases of sexual violence, where verbal testimony frequently serves as pivotal evidence or its corroborative element, supporting and validating other forms of evidence (Menaker and Cramer 2012). As stated at the outset of the article, EN dismissed numerous women's testimonies as unclear, incomprehensible, and lacking credibility, and did not always secure medical aid for its charges. For example, 26-year-old Lea Jakobovitz, initially identified by EN as requiring specialised medical care, encountered difficulties in hospital admission. During her visits to EN's offices, she expressed concerns about neighbours conspiring to sell her to traffickers. Her relatives reported a decline in her mental health over the past three years, during which she believed her brothers were colluding with individuals exploiting her. Initially, EN provided reassurance and promised protection. In subsequent visits, her distress escalated, with EN describing her as having 'a haggard face and profound signs of suffering'. On her third visit, she energetically pleaded for protection from'persistent enemies'. Despite Lea's repeated appeals and requests for EN's assistance, she was not granted a medical examination or hospitalisation. EN later discovered that she was entangled in what they termed an 'unhappy love affair' (CAHJP, AR/EN-3590, *Memoria de la 'Ezras Noshim' de Buenos Aires. Año 1936*, 54–66). Based on the case details, it seems that Lea Jakobovitz's situation may have been trivialised, meaning its seriousness was underestimated despite her evident and ongoing distress. The way she expressed her fears and needs might have been misunderstood. If EN interpreted her emotional turmoil as stemming from personal issues such as romantic relationships, or perhaps even attributed it to her own faults, rather than recognising it as a genuine threat or urgent need for protection, this could have led to inadequate attention and support for her situation.

There is an extensive and growing body of work on testimonies in which an individual experiences injustice specifically in relation to their role as a perceiver or knowledge holder. A contemporary perspective on 'epistemic injustice' comes from British philosopher Miranda Fricker, who coined the term. She introduced 'testimonial injustice' where a speaker unjustly faces a credibility deficit due to prejudice from the listener (Fricker 2007, 17–22), and 'hermeneutical injustice', exemplified when individuals, particularly women in cases of sexual abuse, struggle to fully grasp and articulate their experiences, resulting in communication perceived as unintelligible to others (Ibid., 159–160). The correlation between EN's initial assessment of testimonies and the concept of epistemic injustice implies a recurring pattern where women's narratives may have been disregarded or undermined, presenting an additional challenge in expressing experiences, particularly those involving sexual violence. Fricker emphasises the significance of this concept in historical contexts, noting that terms like 'sexual harassment' only surfaced later in the twentieth century, potentially hindering women from articulating their experiences earlier due to a lack of appropriate vocabulary (Ibid., 6).

Concluding a general approach to cases handled by EN proves challenging, given the complexities and nuanced nature of each situation. It is conceivable that certain EN social workers may have internalised dismissive perceptions, potentially directed towards women or even specifically Jewish women. Some injustices appear more systematic, while others, as Fricker suggests, may be incidental (Ibid., 156–159). The potential biases of EN's staff, whether conscious or unconscious, could have exacerbated the marginalisation of the already vulnerable group. While EN's records mention the names of the organisation's executive members, they do not provide any information about their personal and professional background, training, or suitability for the role. Moreover, EN's communications with the London office show that the organisation was in serious debt in the 1930s (University of Southampton, Special Collection, MS 173, Archives of Jewish Care, 2/5/4, *Minutes of the Finance Committee*, 179–181, 368). The unstable political and financial conditions likely led to inconsistent case management and support. As the organisation continued to evolve, systematic responses and clear protocols may not have been fully established resulting in some of EN's charges not receiving adequate attention.[7]

[7] I was unable to locate evidence of clear case management protocols in the archive.

## 6 Reassessing Historical Narratives of Sex Work and Sexual Violence

The massive and global movement of people, coupled with increasing poverty and hunger in Europe, limited working opportunities, and the concentration of men in specific regions, who often migrated first before their families joined them, led some Jews and other migrants to turn to sex work as a means of survival. Buenos Aires emerged as a hub for the sex trade, aided by its regulated prostitution system from 1875 to the mid-1930s.[8] The presumed hypervisibility of Jewish men in organised sex work activities alarmed global Jewish communities, who feared social stigma and immigration restrictions. In response, these communities distanced themselves from those involved in the Jewish sex work industry by promoting the 'white slavery' narrative, which depicted Jewish women as innocent, naïve, inexperienced, and victimised by unscrupulous procurers (Bristow 1982; Mirelman 1984). Scholars generally agree that the prevalence of trafficking cases labelled as 'white slavery' was exaggerated and the portrayal of women as gullible and unsuspecting overstated (Doezema 1999; Walkowitz 1992; Yarfitz 2020, 6). This has led many historians, influenced by feminist perspectives, to approach the topic and the use of terms like 'prostitution' and 'sex work' with caution, recognising their complex and contested meanings (García 2014). Emphasising the term 'sex worker' in historical analysis may imply a recognition of agency and decision-making abilities attributed to those involved in the exchange of sexual activities for compensation (Orchard 2020). The word 'prostitution' is frequently associated with pejorative connotations, including moral disapproval and links to criminality. Some contend that prostitution inherently involves sexual violence, as it entails exploitation, manipulation, and a lack of genuine consent (Musto et al 2015, 281–282). Despite this, the term is often employed in historical analyses more neutrally to capture the language and attitudes of the

[8] From 1875 prostitution was regulated by the establishment of brothels, the registration and taxation of prostitutes, and the implementation of regular medical check-ups for them. In 1934 regulated prostitution in Buenos Aires ceased, and in 1936 Argentina enacted its nationwide anti-venereal prophylaxis law, marking the definitive end of regulated prostitution across the country.

period under study, offering insights into how societies of the past represented the subject, even as contemporary perspectives on it continue to change.

In my research, I usually highlight the concept of agency to provide more complex narratives of historical sex workers, recognising their autonomy and individual choices. However, I am aware that focusing exclusively on the notion of agency can inadvertently downplay or overlook instances of forced prostitution and sexual violence. Therefore, while I strive to deconstruct binary narratives about the history of prostitution—moving beyond simplistic views that either romanticise or vilify sex work—I must also be vigilant not to dismiss or minimise the experiences of those who endured trafficking or coercion. Paradoxically, reading the archives 'against the grain' (Stoler 2009) in this context involves being aware of how current perspectives on these issues might influence our critique and judgment of historical approaches to handling sexual violence cases. For example, EN reported the case of Esther Blumenthal, who arrived in Buenos Aires at the age of 22. Initially working as a seamstress and living with her relatives, Esther was supported by them as 'they sought to shield her from the potential dangers young women might face without work'. For two years, her life seemed stable, but this changed dramatically when she became involved with a 'dishonourable man' who seduced her and then abandoned her upon discovering she was pregnant. Esther concealed her pregnancy from her family, but once they found out, they disowned her, leaving her without support. In her despair, she attempted suicide. A family, likely not her own, intervened and took her in, offering a modest income in exchange for domestic work. This arrangement lasted nearly a year. EN observed that Esther's intense emotional suffering deeply scarred her, diminishing her will and self-confidence. She began associating with men 'freely', which resulted in what the report describes as her 'complete degradation'. EN suggested that her only hope was to find a man who could marry her and help her improve her life (CAHJP, AR/EN 3590, *Memoria de la 'Ezras Noshim' de Buenos Aires. Año 1936*, 8–10).

Esther Blumenthal's case can be interpreted as involving aspects of sexual violence. Her interaction with a 'dishonourable man'—presumably a procurer—reveals a significant power imbalance, potential manipulation, and deceit. The profound impact of this abandonment, pregnancy out of wedlock, familial rejection, and subsequent suicide attempt underscores the severity of the emotional turmoil she faced, which can be viewed as a form of violence. Although Esther's later involvement in sex work, which EN described as 'a lack of qualms about interacting with men' (Ibid., 10), was not necessarily inherently sexually violent, it likely stemmed from earlier experiences of emotional coercion. Systemic issues and underlying root causes play a role in how sexual violence occurs, manifests, and persists over time. EN and others believed that securing employment and/or finding a husband would improve Esther's situation and enhance her mental well-being. However, this approach may not have fully addressed the long-term consequences of her past experiences or the ongoing impact of sexual violence's perpetuation.

## 7 Next Station: Callao-Raquel Liberman

Upon my return to Buenos Aires in 2024, I anticipate disembarking at the very central station called *Callao*, soon to be renamed *Callao-Raquel Liberman* (Zunino 2023). This upcoming change in station nomenclature symbolises a bridge between historical narratives and contemporary efforts to confront and address issues of exploitation and harassment. It is just one among numerous ways to honour Liberman, who is already extensively featured in Argentine media, television, and literature. For example, Myrtha Schalom wrote a bestselling novel titled *La Polaca* (Schalom 2013). The term *la polaca* is a colloquial expression in Argentina used to refer to a prostitute, but it also literally means a Polish woman, often implying a Polish–Jewish woman (Guy 1995, 54). Liberman's story has also been prominently featured in popular culture. The recent Argentine telenovela *Argentina, Tierra de Amor y Venganza*, which translates into English as 'Argentina, Land of Love and Vengeance', incorporates aspects of her story into its central plot (Bauso 2019).

In 1922, Liberman arrived in Argentina with her children to reunite with her husband, who had already travelled to the country. Soon widowed and facing serious financial challenges, she turned to prostitution, either coerced or by choice, working for the *Zwi Migdal*, a Jewish group engaged in pimping in South America during the early twentieth century (Yarfitz, 2019, 79–95). Having saved sufficient funds, Raquel eventually left the brothel and opened an antique shop. Concerned that her success could serve as a precedent for other prostitutes, the *Zwi Migdal* began harassing Raquel and seizing her belongings. Not being able to successfully face these challenges, she married a procurer, and endured exploitation, ultimately seeking help from the Argentine police.

Her testimony led to the conviction of some of the traffickers, making her a symbol of victimised women and raising awareness about forced prostitution (Glickman 2000, 43–46).

Contemporary media frequently depicts Raquel Liberman as a victim of deception and exploitation, with only a few exceptions deviating from this portrayal (Butierrez and Yarfitz 2023). While her story shares some commonalities with the traditional 'white slavery' narrative, it also significantly diverges from it. Unlike many accounts within this narrative, Raquel did not enter Argentina through a trafficking network nor was she married under a so-called *shtile khupe*, a term derived from the Yiddish for a 'quiet *chuppah* (canopy)/wedding', a practice where a Jewish wedding was performed without the presence of a rabbi, and featuring a prenuptial agreement with one of the traffickers or pimps already listed as the groom (Yarfitz 2020, 3–6). The exact circumstances that led her into prostitution remain largely unknown, adding a layer of mystery to her story. Despite these uncertainties, Raquel's narrative is marked by a degree of agency as she managed to attain financial independence through her work in the sex trade (Glickman 2000, 46). Moreover, unlike other women associated with *Ezras Noshim*, whose identities are often protected for privacy, Raquel's name has always been and remains widely recognised. This widespread recognition has turned her into a symbolic figure representing all victims of sexual violence, though her own story is far from straightforward. The simplified narrative that often circulates in the media fails to capture the full complexity of her life, yet it has been instrumental in gaining publicity for advocacy and support organisations.

In 2011, the city of Buenos Aires inaugurated the Raquel Liberman Award, which is presented every two years to organisations promoting and safeguarding the rights of women who experience violence (Igualdad de Género 2019). The most recent winner was *Madres Víctimas de Trata* (Mothers of Trafficking Victims), an organisation made up of a collective comprising mothers, family members, friends, volunteers, artists, and allies of trafficked women and children (Barriada 2023). Nominations in recent years have included organisations working with survivors of child abuse (Derechos Humanos BA 2021), with the trans community, those offering work and education opportunities, and anti-trafficking advocacy organisations. One recently nominated organisation is *Shalom Bait* (Peace at Home) which provides legal, medical, and psycho-social support to women and children experiencing gender-based violence and abuse. On their website, *Shalom Bait* observes that gender-based violence within the Jewish community 'was an issue very few people wanted to discuss; it remained hidden, in the privacy of the home. The fact of belonging to a minority, a gregarious social group, and with a history of persecution, contributes to keeping problems 'inside'. By denying their existence, the victims are also denied' (Shalom Bait n.d.). *Shalom Bait*'s statement underscores how minority communities sometimes hide certain issues, particularly those related to sexual behaviours. Organisations that cater to specific minority, ethnic, or religious groups may aim to shield the community from external scrutiny, as we have seen above in the case of EN, which was set up partly to counter associations between the Jewish community and the sex trade.

Similarly, organisations supporting victims and survivors of gender-based violence often resort to oversimplified narratives to enhance resources, gain recognition, and raise public awareness (Baker 2018). This was also the case in the 1930s. By amplifying narratives of victimisation and trafficking, EN aimed to mobilise international concerns to secure funding. Although the vocal advocacy of both the global and local Jewish communities may have led to disproportionate attention to Jewish involvement in organised prostitution, thereby unintentionally reinforcing stereotypes and scrutiny, the funding garnered from aligning with simplified narratives relating to exploitation and 'white slavery' allowed EN to broaden its initiatives. In so doing, EN was able to produce and preserve records that offer insights into various facets of Jewish life in Argentina and beyond in the early-to-mid twentieth century.

## 8 Conclusion

Working with the *Ezras Noshim* archives, and the cases contained therein, exemplifies the challenges faced by researchers exploring historical sexual violence. In EN's reports, evidence of sexual violence may be subtle, concealed, or obscured by the environment and circumstances in which they were created. The complexity of interpreting terms like, for example, 'mental illness with a sexual origin', highlights the need for context-sensitive analysis. This type of analysis must account for the inherent limitations of historical records, the subjective nature of historical interpretation, and difficulties in tracing the lived experiences of women whose voices were mediated through institutional and communal lenses.

While EN's efforts to provide medical care and general support are evident, their approach also reflects broader societal attitudes towards women that could be dismissive or stigmatising. The terminology and concepts we use today, such as 'sexual violence' and 'sex work' may not perfectly align with past realities, yet they remain crucial for unpacking the power dynamics and societal pressures of the period under study. The concept of epistemic injustice also proves useful, as it helps us to understand both the challenges women encountered in articulating their experiences and the potential biases of those receiving and listening to their accounts. Generalising EN's approach is challenging because each woman's case illustrates the tailored nature of the organisation's responses and the absence of more standardised frameworks and procedures. Nevertheless, it appears that EN did not aim to isolate the women who sought their help. Instead, their primary focus was on providing prompt treatment to enable quick recovery and reintegration into society. While this focus on rapid reintegration was well-intentioned, it risked overlooking the potential for negative lasting impacts on women's mental health. However, the approach taken by EN should be assessed with an awareness of the constraints the organisation faced, in particular their limited resources, and the broader context in which understandings of the longer-term impacts of sexual violence were not yet well understood.

Finally, the chapter advocates for a broader use of community archives and alternative sources to enhance our comprehension of historical sexual violence and inform current discussions on the subject. It calls for more nuanced representations of sexual violence, moving beyond oversimplified narratives that, while sometimes useful for mobilising advocacy and organisational resources, may not fully capture the complexity of the issue. While this chapter has focused on traces of sexual violence and medicalisation within the EN archives, the records hold promise for examining gender-based violence more broadly. Future areas for empirical research that are potentially fruitful include domestic abuse, other forms of structural and interpersonal violence, and their impact on victims, survivors, and their potential descendants. Thus, community archives are a promising, and underused resource through which to examine questions of the intersection between gender-based violence, medicine, psychiatry, and broader societies.

**Funding** The chapter is part of a doctoral project funded by a fellowship from the Department of Archaeology, History, Cultural Studies, and Religion at the University of Bergen. The author declares no competing interests.

# References

## Primary Sources

Central Archives for the History of the Jewish People (CAHJP), Jerusalem, Israel.
AR/EN-3590.
AR/EN-3960.
University of Southampton Special Collections, Southampton, United Kingdom.
MS 173, Archives of Jewish Care.

## Secondary Sources

Ablard, Jonathan. D. 2008. *Madness in Buenos Aires: Patients, Psychiatrists, and the Argentinian State, 1880–1983*. Calgary: University of Calgary Press.

Ablard, Jonathan D. 2009. The Limits of Psychiatric Reform in Argentina, 1890–1946. In *The Confinement of the Insane: International Perspectives, 1800–1965*, ed. Roy Porter and David Wright, 226–247. Cambridge: Cambridge University Press.

Armus, Diego. 2019. Desirable and Undesirable Migrants. Disease, Eugenics, and Discourses in Modern Buenos Aires. *Journal of Iberian and Latin American Studies* 25: 57–79.

Avni, Haim. 2014. *Clientes, rufianes y prostitutas. Comunidades judias de Argentina e Israel frente a la trata de blancas*. Buenos Aires: Editorial Leviatan.

Baker, Alice. 2018. *Responding to the Forgotten Victims: Examining the Employment of Simplified Narratives by Civil Society Organizations Responding to Conflict-Related Sexual Violence Perpetrated Against Men in Northern Uganda*. Unpublished MA Thesis, Utrecht University.

Bjerg, Maria. 2016. Male Narratives from the Margins of the Country of Immigrants: Two Norwegians in Argentina in the 1920s. In *Expectations Unfulfilled: Norwegian Migrants in Latin America, 1820–1940*, ed. Steinar A. Sæther, 162–183. Leiden: Brill.

Bourke, Joanna. 2012. Sexual Violence, Bodily Pain, and Trauma: A History. *Theory, Culture & Society* 29: 25–51.

Bristow, Edward J. 1982. *Prostitution and Prejudice: The Jewish Fight Against White Slavery, 1870–1939*. Oxford: Clarendon Press.

Bryce, Benjamin. 2015. Paternal Communities: Social Welfare and Immigration in Argentina, 1880–1930. *Journal of Social History* 49: 213–236.

Bryce, Benjamin, and David M.K.. Sheinin. 2017. *Making Citizens in Argentina*. Pittsburgh, PA: University of Pittsburgh Press.

Deutsch, Sandra McGee. 2010. *Crossing Borders, Claiming a Nation: A History of Argentine Jewish Women, 1880–1955*. London: Duke University Press.

Doezema, Jo 1999. Loose Women or Lost Women? The Re-emergence of the Myth of White Slavery in Contemporary Discourses of Trafficking in Women. *Gender Issues* 18: 23–50.

Dovio, Mariana. 2012. Representaciones sobre mujeres de 'mala vida' en Revista Archivos de Psiquiatría, Criminología, Medicina Legal y Ciencias Afines y Revista de Criminología, Psiquiatría y Medicina Legal (1902–1935). In *Mujeres en cuestión: Escrituras, ideologías y cuerpos*, ed. Silvina Beatriz Barroso, Mariana Dovio, López Tessore, Verónica Lucia, and Maria Ignacia Giannoni, 97–140. Buenos Aires: Teseo.

Fricker, Miranda. 2007. *Epistemic Injustice: Power and the Ethics of Knowing*. Oxford: Oxford University Press.

García, Magaly Rodríguez. 2014. Prostitution in World Cities (1600s-2000s). In *Reframing Prostitution: From Discourse to Description, From Moralization to Normalization*, ed. Nina Peršak and Gert Vermeulen, 25–51. Antwerp: Maklu.

Germani, Gino. 1966. Mass Immigration and Modernization in Argentina. *Studies in Comparative International Development* 2: 165–182.

Glickman, Nora. 2000. *The Jewish White Slave Trade and the Untold Story of Raquel Liberman*. New York: Garland.

Glowacka, Dorota. 2021. Sexual Violence Against Men and Boys During the Holocaust: A Genealogy of (Not-So-Silent) Silence. *German History* 39: 78–99.

Golcman, Alejandra. 2017. *El trabajo clinico psiquiátrico en el Buenos Aires del Siglo XX*. Madrid: Catarata.

Gordon, David M. 2018. Reading the Archives as Sources. In *Oxford Research Encyclopedia of African History*. https://doi.org/10.1093/acrefore/9780190277734.013.227

Granick, Jaclyn. 2021. *International Jewish Humanitarianism in the Age of the Great War*. Cambridge: Cambridge University Press.

Grey, Daniel J.R., and Eliza Teixeira de Toledo. 2022. Histories of Sexual Violence in Nineteenth and Twentieth Century Latin America: An Introduction. *Historia Critica* 86: 3–16.

Guy, Donna J. 1995. *Sex and Danger in Buenos Aires: Prostitution, Family and Nation in Argentina*. London: University of Nebraska Press.

Guy, Donna J. 2009. *Women Build the Welfare State: Performing Charity and Creating Rights in Argentina, 1880–1955*. Durham: Duke University Press.

Hájková, Anna. 2022. Why We Need a History of Prostitution in the Holocaust. *European Review of History: Revue Européenne D'histoire* 29: 194–222.

Hart, Mitchell B. 2007. *The Healthy Jew: The Symbiosis of Judaism and Modern Medicine*. Cambridge: Cambridge University Press.

Heberle, Renée J. 2014. Sexual Violence. In *The Oxford Handbook of Gender, Sex, and Crime*, ed. Rosemary Gartner and Bill McCarthy, 59–76. Oxford: Oxford University Press.

Hedgepeth, Sonja M., and Rochelle G. Saidel, eds. 2010. *Sexual Violence Against Jewish Women During the Holocaust*. Waltham, MA: Brandeis University Press.

Kałczewiak, Mariusz. 2019. *Polish Jews, Interwar Migration, and the Emergence of Transatlantic Jewish Culture*. Tuscaloosa: University of Alabama Press.

Knepper, Paul. 2007. 'Jewish Trafficking' and London Jews in the Age of Migration. *Journal of Modern Jewish Studies* 6: 239–256.

Lammasniemi, Laura. 2024. Capacity to Consent to Sex: A Historical Perspective. *Oxford Journal of Legal Studies*. https://doi.org/10.1093/ojls/gqae029

Lesser, Jeffrey. 1995. *Welcoming the Undesirables: Brazil and the Jewish Question*. Berkeley: University of California Press.

Lesser, Jeffrey, and Raanan Rein. 2008. *Rethinking Jewish-Latin Americans*. Albuquerque, NM: University of New Mexico Press.

Menaker, Tasha A., and Robert J. Cramer. 2012. The Victim as Witness: Strategies for Increasing Credibility Among Rape Victim-Witnesses in Court. *Journal of Forensic Psychology Practice* 12: 424–438.

Mirelman, Victor A. 1984. The Jewish Community Versus Crime: The Case of White Slavery in Buenos Aires. *Jewish Social Studies* 46: 145–168.

Musto, Jennifer, Crystal A. Jackson, and E. Shih. 2015. Prostitution and Sex Work. In *International Encyclopedia of the Social & Behavioral Sciences*, 2nd ed., ed. James D. Wright, 279–285. Amsterdam: Elsevier.

Orchard, Treena. 2020. Sex Work and Prostitution. In *Encyclopedia of Sexuality and Gender*, ed. A. Lykins. Cham: Springer. https://doi.org/10.1007/978-3-319-59531-3_15-1.

Person, Katarzyna. 2015. Sexual Violence During the Holocaust: The Case of Forced Prostitution in the Warsaw Ghetto. *Shofar* 33: 103–121.

Reggiani, Andrés H. 2010. Depopulation, Fascism, and Eugenics in 1930s Argentina. *The Hispanic American Historical Review* 90: 283–318.

Rodriguez, Julia. 2006. *Civilizing Argentina: Science, Medicine, and the Modern State*. Chapel Hill: University of North Carolina Press.

Schalom, Myrtha. 2013. *La polaca*. Buenos Aires: Galerna.

Schettini, Cristiana. 2017. A Social History of Prostitution in Buenos Aires. In *Selling Sex in the City: A Global History of Prostitution, 1600s-2000s*, ed. Magaly Rodríguez García, Lex Heerma van Voss and Elise van Nederveen Meerkerk, 357–85. Leiden: Brill.

Stadler, Lelia. 2020. In Search of Wandering Husbands: Jewish Migration, Desertion, and Divorce Between Poland and Argentina, 1919–1939. In *Migrants, Refugees, and Asylum Seekers in Latin America*, ed. Raanan Rein, Stefan Rinke, and David. M.K. Sheinin, 17–44. Leiden: Brill.

Stepan, Nancy. 1991. *The Hour of Eugenics: Race, Gender, and Nation in Latin America*. Ithaca, NY: Cornell University Press.
Stoler, Ann Laura. 2009. *Along the Archival Grain: Epistemic Anxieties and Colonial Common Sense*. Princeton, NJ: Princeton University Press.
Walkowitz, Judith R. 1992. *City of Dreadful Delight: Narratives of Sexual Danger in Late-Victorian London*. Chicago: University of Chicago Press.
Wright, David, and Renée Saucier. 2012. Madness in the Archives: Anonymity, Ethics, and Mental Health History Research. *Journal of the Canadian Historical Association* 23: 65–90.
Wyers, Mark David. 2017. Coercion and Voluntarism in Sex Work. In *Selling Sex in the City: A Global History of Prostitution, 1600s-2000s*, ed. Magaly Rodríguez García, Lex Heerma van Voss and Elise van Nederveen Meerkerk, 775–800. Leiden: Brill.
Yarfitz, Mir. 2013. Uprooting the Seeds of Evil: Ezras Noschim and Jewish Marriage Regulation, Morality Certificates, and Degenerate Prostitute Mothers in 1930s Buenos Aires. In *The New Jewish Argentina: Facets of Jewish Experience in the Southern Cone*, ed. Adriana Brodsky and Raanan Rein, 55–79. Leiden: Brill.
Yarfitz, Mir. 2019. *Impure Migration: Jews and Sex Work in Golden Age Argentina*. New Brunswick: Rutgers University Press.
Yarfitz, Mir. 2020. Marriage as Ruse or Migration Route: Jewish Women's Mobility and Sex Trafficking to Argentina, 1890s-1930s. *Women in Judaism: A Multidisciplinary E-Journal*, 17: https://doi.org/10.33137/wij.v17i1.34964

## Online Sources

Barriada. 2023. Madres Víctimas de Trata ganó el Premio Raquel Liberman. Barriada, 23 September. https://www.barriada.com.ar/madres-victimas-de-trata-gano-el-premio-raquel-liberman. Accessed 1 January 2024.
Bauso, Matías. 2019. La dura vida de Raquel Liberman: La prostituta polaca que inspiró a la China Suárez y se convirtió en un símbolo de la lucha contra la trata. Infobae, 25 March. https://www.infobae.com/sociedad/2019/03/25/la-dura-vida-de-raquel-liberman-la-prostituta-polaca-que-inspiro-a-la-china-suarez-y-se-convirtio-en-un-simbolo-de-la-lucha-contra-la-trata. Accessed 1 January 2024.
Buenos Aires Government. 2019. El Gobierno porteño, contra el acoso callejero. https://buenosaires.gob.ar/noticias/el-gobierno-porteno-contra-el-acoso-callejero. Accessed 1 January 2024.

Butierrez, M. J., and M. Yarfitz. 2023. Una mirada crítica sobre la estación Callao-Raquel Liberman. Latfem, 25 September. https://latfem.org/una-mirada-critica-sobre-la-estacion-callao-raquel-liberman. Accessed 27 December 2023.

Derechos Humanos BA. 2021. Organizaciones postuladas - Premio Raquel Liberman 2021 https://www.youtube.com/watch?v=NXYbqNS1OEM. Accessed 15 January 2024.

Igualdad de Género. 2019. Premio Raquel Liberman. Buenos Aires Ciudad. https://buenosaires.gob.ar/noticias/premio-raquel-liberman. Accessed 21 December 2023.

Shalom Bait. n.d. ¿Quiénes somos? Shalom Bait. https://www.shalombait.org.ar/en/quienes-somos. Accessed 1 January 2024.

Zunino, Daiana. 2023. Subte: El emotivo nombre con el que rebautizarán la estación Callao de la línea D. La Nación, September 7. https://www.lanacion.com.ar/sociedad/subte-el-emotivo-nombre-con-el-que-rebautizaran-la-estacion-callao-de-la-linea-d-nid07092023. Accessed 1 January 2024.

# ‘We Are Not Inclined To Accept the Rape Story’: Medical Evidence and Sexual Violence in Kenya, c.1920–1960

*Rhian Elinor Keyse*

## 1 Introduction

On 31 January 1943, an unnamed fifteen-year-old Kikuyu girl was found injured beside the railway line near Kijabe, central Kenya. She was taken to Kijabe Mission Hospital, and from there to Kikuyu Mission Hospital, where she remained a patient for several weeks. Police assumed that she had fallen from a moving train. However, over a month later, when she recovered sufficiently to give a statement, the teenager gave the police a more troubling account of her injuries. She described how after joining the train, 7 African soldiers pulled her into a compartment and raped her before throwing her out of the carriage. Yet, even before this disclosure, medical staff suspected she had been sexually assaulted. The Sister-in-Charge at Kijabe tried to examine her for evidence of rape on admission but was ‘prevented from doing so by the complainant’, and did not pass on her concerns when the girl was transferred. In the absence of corroborative medical evidence, no positively identified assailants, and

R. E. Keyse (✉)
University of Wales Trinity Saint David, Carmarthen, UK
e-mail: r.keyse@uwtsd.ac.uk


R. E. Keyse et al. (eds.), *Sexual Violence in Medicine and Psychiatry*, Genders and Sexualities in History,
https://doi.org/10.1007/978-3-032-10800-5_10

under pressure from superior officers to reduce resources allocated to the case, Mr. Griffiths, Assistant Superintendent of the Railway and Harbour Police, reported that 'we are not inclined to accept the rape story'. Despite the Sister-in-Charge's initial suspicions that the girl had been raped, Griffiths speculated that the attending doctor appeared 'sceptical about her story although he has not actually said so'. With the girl's reluctance to engage with medical examination taken as evidence of mendacity, Griffiths concluded that the story was 'fabricated'. The girl had, he opined, likely alighted from the moving train to avoid walking four miles to her employers' home, but misjudged the train's speed and invented the rape to explain her injuries. The enquiry was closed shortly thereafter (Kenya National Archives [henceforth KNA] AM/1/5).

This fragmentary insight into an alleged assault raises key issues facing survivors of sexual violence as they navigated colonial medico-legal systems in Kenya: delayed or absent medical examinations; lack of communication between medical professionals; and survivors' reluctance to engage with medical examinations. It also hints at the meanings investigating authorities attached to medical evidence and survivors' responses. These are not just historical issues. In contemporary Kenya, an estimated 15.2% of women have experienced sexual violence (National Crime Research Centre 2015). The recent Covid-19 pandemic further brought into relief the lack of timely medical treatment and psycho-social support for survivors of gender-based violence (Human Rights Watch 2021). Sexual violence services are under-resourced, with survivors often struggling to access forensic examinations and tests (Rockowitz et al 2023; Kilonzo et al. 2009a; 2009b; Wangamati et al. 2021), and forensic evidence is often poorly collected and preserved (Ajema et al 2011; Olson et al 2022; Temmerman et al. 2019). Such obstacles occur in the context of broader healthcare inequalities, exacerbated by barriers such as medical fees, limited transportation, and geographical location of clinics (Muinde and Prince 2023; Ilinca et al. 2019), resulting from historical processes dating to colonial rule (Chirwa 2016). Given these pressing contemporary issues, it is perhaps surprising that historians of sexual violence in Africa have paid little attention to medico-legal responses, despite a growing literature on such violence in colonial contexts (Scully 1995; Benson and Chadya 2005; Shadle 2008; Thornberry 2019; Reuther 2018), the wide literature on histories of medicine in Africa (Vaughan 1991; Lee 2021), and emerging histories of forensic medicine in other contexts (Jentzen 2019; Kolsky 2010; Singh 2021; Wright 2023). This chapter brings together these literatures and historicises these issues by exploring the experiences of women and girls as they navigated colonial medico-legal structures in the aftermath of assault, as well as the uses and meanings of medical evidence in colonial courtrooms. It argues that medical responses to sexual violence in colonial Kenya were rooted in the logics of a racially stratified settler colony, with practical and ideological effects. The segregated healthcare system, and unequal investment in infrastructure, meant that 'Native' patients received lower quality care than their 'European' counterparts. Moreover, colonial logics inherent in responses to sexual violence went beyond the bricks-and-mortar availability of clinics and physicians, with medico-legal evidence serving to produce and reproduce gendered, classed and racialised knowledge about victims and survivors. This chapter therefore builds on Shadle's (2008) important corrective to the idea that African culture uniquely oppresses women, which demonstrated that customary courts in colonial Gusiiland were often more sympathetic to African women complainants than colonial courts, by elucidating how medico-legal 'expertise' was used to shape the racialised and gendered operation of colonial courts, often to the detriment of African women (cf. Sowemimo 2023).

## 2 Sources and Context

Historians have noted the fragmentary nature of archival sources dealing with sexual violence, and the methodological 'foraging' required to reveal their traces (Mertens 2023). This is true of the records drawn on for this chapter. Evidence about historical sexual violence in colonial Kenya is patchy. Official statistical returns are inconsistently categorised, making it difficult to ascertain the extent of reported sexual violence and conviction rates (e.g. Government and Colony of Kenya 1927, 1930). The picture is complicated by the legal pluralism operating in colonial Kenya. Although rape was a capital crime from 1926 to 1955, rendering it theoretically triable only in the Supreme Court of Kenya, in practice cases were often settled out of court by elders or heard in local tribunals, reflecting racialised European assumptions that intra-African rape was not a serious crime, and the concomitant desire of administrators to avoid the resource burden of investigation (Shadle 2008). The existence of other means of recourse mean that colonial court records are necessarily partial (Cooper, 1997, 20–39), while local tribunal records for much of Kenya appear to have been destroyed (Shadle 2008). In addition, Kenyan colonial authorities acknowledged underreporting: Thomas Stanley Ebblewhite, a Crown Prosecutor, noted in 1947 that there had been a 'series' of multiple-perpetrator rape cases. Twelve were under investigation, but others went 'unreported because the women victims are afraid' (KNA AC/2/637).

The chapter is based upon archival material from the period between 1920 and 1960, relating to 84 cases of sexual violence held in the Kenya National Archives (KNA), and drawn from records at different levels of colonial administration; from district police and administrative correspondence to cases heard at the Supreme Court and the East African Court of Appeal (EACA). Victims and survivors have been anonymised through the assignation of initials. The archival record of cases is incomplete, with varying levels of documentation retained in the available case files: some files contain full medical reports, while others include only passing reference to medical evidence. Despite these limitations, colonial legal sources are among the best forms of evidence for investigating the role of medical professionals and ideas in colonial sexual violence cases. As Shadle (2008, 36) notes, medical evidence was more likely to be present in cases heard in colonial than in customary courts. In addition, the way cases were heard at the Supreme Court, with a judge presiding over the trial assisted by African assessors (usually local male elders) charged with advising him on local custom, meant that sometimes African views on medical ideas are accessible, albeit filtered through an elite male lens and colonial court recording.

The cases examined relate to offences of rape, attempted rape, indecent assault, and defilement, as well as murder cases where sexual violence was involved. Until 1930, the law of sexual offences in Kenya was governed by the Indian Penal Code (IPC), as amended by the Criminal Law Amendment Ordinance of 1913. Rape was punishable by a term of up to 14 years'imprisonment, with or without a fine (Barth et al. 1926, 733). Attempted rape attracted up to 10 years' imprisonment, with or without a fine, while the use of criminal force with 'intent to outrage modesty' saw up to 7 years' imprisonment. Defilement, punishable by up to 2 years' imprisonment, could only be committed against a 'white woman under the age of sixteen years' in circumstances which did not amount to rape or attempted rape (Barth et al. 1926, p. 734). The amended IPC further specified that rape cases where a 'native' man was alleged to have assaulted a 'non-native' woman were triable by the Supreme Court (Barth et al. 1926, 735). In 1926, a high-profile case of assault on a white woman inflamed moral panic about the sexual threat to white women from African men, known as 'Black Peril'. Rape was consequently made a capital offence. Ostensibly, the increased punishment applied regardless of race, but in practice the law was applied in heavily racialised ways (Anderson 2010).

The Penal Code of Kenya, introduced in 1930, defined rape as 'unlawful carnal knowledge of a woman or girl, without her consent', or where consent had been obtained by force, threats, intimidation, false representations or impersonation (Kingdon 1948, 218). Indecent assault was punishable by up to 14 years' imprisonment, with consent not being a defence in cases where the girl was under sixteen, unless the accused had reasonable cause to believe that she was sixteen or older (Kingdon 1948). The racial specification for defilement disappeared in the 1930 Penal Code, with the crime now defined as unlawful carnal knowledge of a girl aged under sixteen. Defilement was punishable with life imprisonment, while attempted defilement attracted a prison sentence of up to 14 years. (Kingdon 1948).

## 3 Accessing Medical Care: Survivors' Experiences

The vignette with which this chapter opened raises questions about Kenyan women's experiences of medico-legal interventions after sexual assault, and the barriers they faced in securing corroborative medical evidence. Of course, archival sources are a snapshot of these women's experiences (Bridger and Hazan 2022), mediated through state institutions. As such, we have little insight into their lives before or after the violence they experienced (Fuentes 2016). Nonetheless, certain key themes emerge from the archives.

One persistent issue in archival accounts is delayed examinations for African women and girls complaining of assault. In the case of OA, a child who complained of rape in October 1938, Kericho Medical Officer (MO) Wilkinson found evidence of recent penetration but no bruising, noting that this was not unusual given that there were five days between the alleged offence and his examination (KNA AC/2/311). OA testified that she, her father and uncle had initially reported the assault to their local Assistant Chief Abok. Here began the navigation of several layers of colonial bureaucracy. Abok sent them to the Chief, Opio, who directed them to the accused's Chief at Kericho. From there they were sent to the British District Commissioner (DC), who finally referred OA for medical examination (KNA AC/2/311). In this case, then, delays were inherent in the ideology of 'indirect rule' that prevailed in interwar British Africa, where colonial authorities attempted to govern through 'traditional' authority structures (Ranger 1993; Mamdani 1996). As discussed above, Native Tribunals were empowered to try certain offences—and often tried rape cases despite their being ostensibly a capital offence triable only in the Supreme Court (Shadle 2008). Local chiefs were therefore often a first port of call in reporting assaults, with women and girls like OA being referred to colonial authorities, sometimes at some distance away, resulting in delays to evidence-gathering and investigation.

Other delays were caused by the distance women and girls had to travel to access medical facilities. MOs were usually based in main District stations in towns. Medical provision in outlying areas increased from the 1920s with the introduction of dispensaries, usually under the charge of African assistants with MOs visiting periodically, with a formally organised system of rural healthcare centres established in 1946 (Crozier 2007; Beck 1981). African staff at dispensaries could not undertake medico-legal duties, which were the preserve of qualified doctors. Women and girls from outlying areas could therefore not count on timely treatment and evidence gathering. This could have tragic consequences, as in the 1953 case of MM who was found lying severely injured near Makueni by Roger Coryndon, an official of the African Settlement Board, having been stabbed during an attempted rape. Despite Coryndon administering first aid, and treatment at the local dispensary, MM tragically died en route to hospital at Machakos (KNA AXM1/8/737).

Delays also occurred where those receiving initial reports did not appreciate the urgency of the situation, perhaps owing to racialised notions which downplayed Africans' reports of pain (Bernault 2007; Landau 1996). On Christmas Day 1946, SS, an eight-year-old Nandi girl, reported to her mother that a man had attempted to rape her before assaulting her vaginally and anally with a stick. They reported to Mr. Outram, the Estate Manager of the European estate where they lived. Outram provided bandages and Dettol and sent the party away. SS died early next morning. Dr. Marathe, Sub-Assistant Surgeon at Kapsabet Hospital who carried out the postmortem, testified that SS 'might have survived if medically treated at once'. (KNA AXM1/8/266). Outram explained that he did not take SS for medical attention because he 'did not realise at the time that the child was in danger of dying—I had no idea it was so serious' (KNA AXM1/8/266), again reflecting prevalent ideas that intra-African sexual assault was not a serious matter (Shadle 2008).

European women and girls do not appear to have experienced such delays, with their case records almost universally suggesting near-immediate access to care. In a 1945 case of attempted defilement of two European girls, aged 2 and 5, by their father's African farmhand, the children's mother took the children for medical examination the same day (KNA AXM1/8/1412). Similarly, GMS, a 63-year-old woman raped during a burglary at her home in Nairobi on 12 November 1949, was discovered by her servants at 6.30am and examined at Nairobi European Hospital by two doctors by 9am. (KNA AXM1/8/367). Some European women, such as WP, raped on 27 February 1928, were examined by doctors known to them (KNA AG/52/392). This prompt access to medical care reflects the racialised nature of the colonial health system. Medical facilities were initially established to cater to European communities; European hospitals received higher subsidies, and town-planning prioritised European needs over those of Africans (Crozier 2007; Vaughan 1991). Infrastructure development was also skewed towards European needs, with the colonial government 'explicitly and continuously attempt[ing] to limit Africans' access to the urban core' (Park 2014, 2; Overton 1987). In comparison, standards in 'Native' hospitals 'almost always lagged behind' (Crozier 2007, 94), and spatial segregation meant that Africans, particularly in rural areas, were relatively poorly served by infrastructure and facilities such as roads and hospitals (Overton, 1987), an inequality exacerbated by the fact that European vehicle ownership outstripped that of the African population (Park 2014; White 1990).

Perhaps owing to this inequality of access, or because of a lack of familiarity with 'European' medicine and the evidentiary requirements of bringing a rape prosecution, some African women did not access colonial medical practitioners but instead were treated by local community medicine practitioners. KK, a pregnant woman, was raped in 1936 by two strangers who broke into her home near Kabarnet as she slept with her three children. Suffering a miscarriage the next day, she was treated by two local men who bled her and gave her an unspecified medicine (KNA AC/2/240). Some women and girls, or their guardians, were reluctant to undergo medical examination. In 1939, 6-year-old OW's mother reported to the elders that her child had been raped. Advised that OW would have to be medically examined to pursue the case in the colonial court, the mother was reluctant, and so, 'owing to [her] unhelpful attitude', the DC for Kavirondo reported that nothing further could be done (KNA DC KSM/1/19/219). In a 1956 case, a rape prosecution failed when the complainant did not attend court. Her guardian had prevented her from being medically examined as to her age, a development the presiding judge referred to as 'not at all helpful (to say the least of it)' (KNA AP/1/1845). While colonial officials complained about such reluctance as non-compliance, or evidence of mendacity (KNA AM/1/5), other interpretations are possible, such as unfamiliarity with European medicine, colonial doctors' lack of sensitivity to local practices (Ndege 2002), parental concerns about exposing daughters' bodies to examination by white men (see Odinga 2001), or other barriers such as distance from medical facilities, as discussed above. It is also important to note here that the necessity for medical evidence to proceed with a case in the colonial court was not shared by local customary courts, where witness testimony was sometimes prioritised over medical reports (Shadle 2008).

The case of SS, discussed earlier, highlights another prevalent issue, that of poor handling of forensic evidence. The slides taken by Dr Marathe during the postmortem examination were damaged in transit and could not be analysed. While the accused, as we have seen, was found guilty of SS's murder, Mr. Justice Bourke's scathing judgement condemned police handling of the evidence, given the destruction of the slides and a lack of clarity around the chain of custody of exhibits (KNA AXM1/8/266). Similarly, while analysing the clothing of NK, whose body was found in a forest at Ainabkoi in July 1944 following her rape and murder, Assistant Government Analyst Harry Nefdt found that suspected seminal stains on her clothing had developed 'heavy mould growths' owing to their storage in 'moist conditions'. Nefdt therefore found the evidence inconclusive, suggesting that mould might have 'disintegrated' the sperm cells (KNA AXM1/8/209).

The bodies of women who had been sexually assaulted and murdered could also be mishandled, rendering it impossible to find forensic evidence of sexual violence. The body of thirteen-year-old OO was taken to hospital at Kisii on 13 March 1949, the day of her rape and murder, but was left to lie for two days until the postmortem. By this point, owing to the climate, she was 'extremely decomposed', causing difficulties with establishing her cause of death (KNA AXM1/8/359). The accused was found guilty of murder at the Supreme Court and sentenced to death but appealed to the EACA. Although this was dismissed, the appeal judges noted the unsatisfactory nature of the delayed postmortem (KNA AXM1/8/359).

## 4 The Uses and Meanings of Medical Evidence in Sexual Offence Cases: Age, Corroboration, and Emotion

Given the fragmented evidence, it is not possible to come to definitive conclusions about whether medical evidence affected conviction rates in colonial Kenya, although scholarship from other criminal contexts suggests there is little correlation (Du Mont and Parnis 2000; Quinlan 2017; Mulla 2014). It is possible, however, to demonstrate how medical evidence was presented and contested in the colonial legal system. Elizabeth Kolsky (2010) notes that, historically, British legal thinking about rape and sexual violence was heavily influenced by views expressed in the so-called 'Hale warning', cited by British judges in cases as late as the 1980s. This dictum, originating with seventeenth-century judge Sir Matthew Hale, stated that rape is 'an accusation easily to be made, hard to be proved, and harder yet to be defended by the party accused' (Hale 1736–9, 634). Accusations of sexual violence were therefore treated with suspicion, and the 'behaviour, character, and body' of women making allegations had to be scrutinised for corroboration (Kolsky 2010, 111). In colonial territories, including Kenya, ideas about the potential untrustworthiness of 'native' testimonies added a racialised dimension (Keyse 2019; Kolsky 2010). Colonised women in Kenya and elsewhere who reported sexual violence were suspected by virtue of both their gender and race, an intersection which Kolsky (2010, 110) refers to as the 'double difference' in the colonial courtroom. In this context, police and colonial courts looked to medical experts—as practitioners of an apparently 'objective' discipline—to corroborate or discount accounts of sexual violence. They examined victims for signs of bodily—and occasionally emotional—injury, as well as scrutinising physical exhibits such as clothing for indications of assault. In so doing, they used 'truth-technologies' (Kolsky 2010, 111) such as medical jurisprudence and blood and semen-stain analysis which had become increasingly important since the late-nineteenth century (Bates 2016).

One use of such evidence was determining a complainant's age. Age was a contentious category across British Africa, particularly in the light of humanitarian concerns about child labour, early marriage, and juvenile delinquency (Shadle 2016; Keyse 2019; Walters 2016; Grier 2004). Defining which children needed protection and intervention vexed missionaries, colonial administrators, and medics alike, especially given that lack of birth registration meant that most girls and young women did not have documentary evidence of age (Walters 2016). Brett Shadle has noted that, from the 1930s, colonial discourses around African childhood shifted in Kenya. Emotional and psychological maturity came to be emphasised over chronological age or physiological development in discussions of readiness for marriage (Shadle 2016). This shift is, however, not evident in the investigation or prosecution of sexual offences in the colonial legal system. Given the legal definition of sexual intercourse with girls under sixteen as 'defilement', chronological age was emphasised. If rape could not be proved—for example in cases where the defence successfully argued that a complainant consented—then a conviction for defilement could still succeed if the girl could be shown to be under sixteen.[1] Age was therefore crucial to prosecutions. In a context where local conceptions of age often centred on the attainment of social milestones such as whether a girl had been initiated, married, or given birth to a child (Ominde 1952; Thomas 2003; Wagner 1949; Southall 1952), and where proof of chronological age was unavailable, physiological development became a proxy, and 'objective' medical expertise its arbiter (Bates 2016). In 1938, the alleged attacker of OA, a girl from Kericho District, was tried at the Supreme Court on charges of rape, defilement, and indecent assault. OA's age is difficult to ascertain from the archival record; her initial complaint placed her at 11 years old, but the Preliminary Inquiry noted she was '9 years old or so'. Her father was uncertain as to her age, offering that she had not begun to menstruate and had been a child 'when the hoppers were here' (KNA AC/2/311), a likely reference to famine-causing locust invasions which ravaged Western Kenya in 1928 and 1931 (Ochieng' 1988). Upon medical examination, Kericho MO Dixon ascertained that OA was 11 years old and dismissed suggestions that she might be sixteen as 'quite impossible', given that she had not yet 'reached puberty'. Although accounts of OA's age varied, medical evidence placed her firmly under the age of sixteen, making sexual intercourse with her a criminal matter. With the claim of rape considered

[1] Sixteen was not the age of consent to sex in all circumstances: there was no age of consent to marriage for African girls in Kenya during the colonial period.

adequately corroborated by other witnesses, her assailant was convicted and sentenced to 6 years' imprisonment with hard labour (KNA AC/2/311.). In a similar 1942 case, NM's assailant was charged with rape, defilement, and indecent assault. Her initial complaint stated she was 7 years old, but in court, her mother did not know her exact age. Instead, she relied on events to state that NM was a small child by 1936 'when the health work was started'. NM herself drew on local conceptions of age depending on initiation rites, stating 'I have not yet been circumcised'. Medical evidence was needed to settle the question, with District MO Kerr finding her to be 'about eight years old', although it is not clear what criteria he applied to reach this conclusion. Kerr testified that NM had a cut on her hymen, consistent with 'at least partial penetration', but he could not say whether it was caused by a penis or a finger. The prosecution entered a *nolle prosequi* on the charge of rape, and the case therefore became one of defilement. The judge found NM's age to be under 16 and her injuries corroborative of her complaint, sentencing her assailant to 3 years' imprisonment with hard labour and 15 strokes of the cane (KNA AC/2/404).

For older girls, especially where consent was at issue, medical evidence as to age was recorded more meticulously, thereby maximising possible charges available to prosecutors. LK, a Mkamba girl, complained in 1946 that a stranger had raped her. LK explained that her assailant, before assaulting her, asked if she would tell her father if he had sexual intercourse with her. LK told the court that she had no understanding of the question. Implicit in LK's answer is the idea that she did not possess the knowledge of sex that would be imparted to her on initiation, thus she was not yet a woman according to local mores (KNA AC/2/558; Middleton and Kershaw 1965; Ngutuku and Okwany 2024). Crucially, LK stated that she did not consent and had struggled to resist. Her alleged assailant, however, contended that she had asked him for money as he was passing by (KNA AC/2/558). Perhaps tapping into contemporaneous concerns about young women's sexual licence and prostitution (White 1990) to inform his defence strategy, he stated that he admonished her that 'only a prostitute' would ask a 'strange man' for money, and that LK then offered to have sex with him for fifty cents, which he paid her after intercourse. With the fact of intercourse undisputed, LK's consent was at the crux of the case, and evidence as to her chronological age was crucial to ensure a conviction if the charge of rape failed. Machakos MO Turner concluded that according to dental examination and her 'breast development, pubic hair, etc.', she was under fifteen (KNA AC/2/558). With this medical evidence in hand, the prosecution argued that even if rape could not be proven, defilement had been clearly established. In the event, two of three assessors agreed that LK had not consented and the offence of rape had been proven. The third assessor, while expressing doubts over consent, accepted that LK was under sixteen. Mr Justice Bourke accepted both medical evidence as to LK's age, and evidence that she had resisted. Convicting her assailant of rape, he imposed a sentence of four years' imprisonment with hard labour (KNA AC/2/558).

When other issues were in question, such as the presence or absence of bodily signifiers or physical evidence of violence, differential interpretations gave lie to claims of scientific objectivity. What constituted scientific proof of sexual violence was not consistent, and practitioners differed in the weight ascribed to particular forms of evidence. As Victoria Bates (2016) reminds us for nineteenth-century British cases, medical practitioners were not divorced from their social milieu, but often reflected and contributed to the development of prevalent views and concerns. As predominantly (lower)-middle class men (Crozier 2007) working in a colony which was racially stratified and a settler society which was deeply anxious about maintaining social—and sexual—boundaries between coloniser and colonised (Shadle 2015; Kennedy 1987; Anderson 2010), it is unsurprising that medical practitioners' evidence in Kenyan sexual violence cases carried racialised, gendered, and classed valences. Women's identities—especially racial and ethnic categorisations and gendered roles such as marital status—were ascribed particular meanings. The intersection can be seen clearly in the case of W, a Kamba woman, who reported that she had been raped on 5 July 1935. Returning from market with her co-wife and another woman from her village, W reported that her group had been accosted by four men near a stream. W was raped by two men, with their co-accused raping the other two women. Examining W four days after the assault, Machakos MO Bell stated that he could find no external evidence of injury. While her vagina was 'slightly swollen', he noted that this was not uncommon in 'a married woman subject to very frequent intercourse' (KNA AC/2/223). Bell drew here on colonial constructions of African men and women having voracious sexual appetites (Hammonds 1997; Decker 2021)—in this case to the point of physical injury—to assert that W's story of sexual assault was not necessarily supported by medical evidence. While Mr Justice

Horne returned a guilty verdict in the case of one of W's attackers, the impact of the assumptions contained in Bell's evidence clearly shaped his view of the case. Sentencing the convicted man to four years' imprisonment, Horne referred to the medical evidence, positing that the lack of corroboration of 'personal injury' could be explained by the fact that W was a married woman. However, he went further, suggesting that most African women did not resist rape, and that W 'as in most cases submitted in being caught and beaten a little'. In making this claim, the colonial court—bolstered by medical claims—negated W's testimony of resistance (KNA AC/2/223), a contrast with customary tribunals which accepted women's resistance to sexual intercourse (Shadle 2008). Similar views were found in another case heard before Horne in the same year. C, a pregnant Lumbwa woman, alleged she had been raped by seven men on 29 June 1935 in a forest near Molo. She stated that she had struggled and shouted, and noted that she 'received no outward marks but my stomach was paining me'. She was examined by Nakuru MO Henderson who stated he had found no corroborative evidence of injury. Henderson stated that in his experience of rape cases, he had 'never found signs of injury on any native woman' because the 'Black woman never puts up a fight' (KNA AC/2/222). WhileHorne found one of her assailants guilty of rape and sentenced him to five years' imprisonment, racialised assumptions in the guise of medical expertise again contradicted women's narratives about their own experience of assault. African women testifying in colonial courts asserted their pain and bodily suffering in the face of medical evidence that asserted their supposed lack of injury and reflected racialised assumptions about African women's lack of capacity to feel pain (Bernault 2007; Landau 1996).

Racialised ideas about sexuality were not limited to cases involving African women and girls. A, a three-year-old Goan girl alleged that an African man had touched her 'private parts' while she was playing on the verandah of her Nairobi home. The man was tried at the Supreme Court in 1928 on a charge of using criminal force to outrage the modesty of a woman. When questioned, A testified that she had 'told him to do this'. Dr Kauntze, the Deputy Director of Laboratory Services at Nairobi who shortly afterwards became editor of the influential *East African Medical Journal* (Ombongi et al. 1998), was called to give evidence about seminal stains on the child's clothing. Kauntze opined about the sexual desires of children of A's age. He said that while he 'couldn't say from my own experience that a child of that age could express a sexual desire', he suggested that 'children of that age do play sexually with one another' (KNA AG/52/390). Although Kauntze was clear that his observation applied to children 'irrespective of race', it is striking that such medical opinion is absent from cases involving European children (see, for example, AG/52/394; AXM1/8/1412). The three African assessors in the case believed that the accused had touched the child but agreed that she may have encouraged him. The accused was acquitted, with Mr Justice Sheridan concluding that for the charge to be proved, the modesty of the child needed to have been outraged, which he argued could not be proved given the child 'invited the accused to do something'. Blaming her mother for letting A out of her sight, Sheridan concluded that 'children will play with each other sexually and this fact alone should...put parents on their guard' (KNA AG/52/390). This decision elicited outrage from the Indian-owned press in Kenya. *The Democrat* published a scathing editorial expressing indignance that 'we are asked to take it for granted by a European judge that a child of this age, not known to be in any way precocious, was sufficiently conscious to have a keen perception of sexual joy and was hardened to it so far as to be dead to all sense of modesty', and decrying the hypocrisy of the colonial state's claims to promote child welfare while a colonial court asked a 'tiny little child...these questions which elicited these woefully innocent replies' (*The Democrat,* 21 January, 1928). While the attribution of sexual precocity to a three-year-old child might seem jarring, it is important to note that A's case was tried just five years after the height of Kenya's 'Indian Crisis' in 1923, a period when Kenyan-Indians were advocating for political equality with Europeans. Elizabeth Williams (2018) notes that gender and sexuality were key to European opposition to Indians' rights claims, arguing that they practised 'deviant sexual behaviours' such as child marriage and premature maternity. Indians' sexual proclivities, according to prominent settlers, rendered them unsuitable to govern Africans, who were considered morally and sexually vulnerable to such deviance. In this sense, then, the notion of an Indian child inciting an African man to sexual behaviour can be read as an extension of such racialised ideas, demonstrating how the colonial court reinforced dominant racialised stereotypes.

The apparent difficulty in proving sexual violence against married women was another feature of cases during this period. F, a Ugandan woman, reported that two men had attacked her on 24 May 1945 as she returned from market near Naivasha. F testified that the first man had intercourse with her against her will while the second man held her by her arms. Naivasha MO Bunny examined F the day after the assault, noting that she had no injury to her vulva and that smears from her vagina were negative for spermatozoa. Bunny therefore reported inconclusive findings, noting that lack of injury was not 'consistent or inconsistent' with rape given that F was married, and that evidence relating to the presence of spermatozoa was inexact and time-sensitive. While spermatozoa could theoretically survive in the vagina for more than 48 hours, he argued that in his experience he would not expect to find them unless smears were taken within five hours of the offence. This demonstrated the contingent and contextual nature of supposedly 'objective' scientific evidence. In the absence of genital injury, other signs on the body could assume more importance. Even though the act of rape itself could not be proved by medical evidence, Bunny noted that F had grazes and scratches on her arms and feet, consistent with her story of being pressed against the ground (KNA AC/2/514). Both accused were convicted and sentenced to 5 years' imprisonment with hard labour and 12 strokes for rape. (*East African Standard* 2 February 1946).

Corroboration operated differently for some European women and girls who sought redress through courts, reflecting views relating to the perceived respectability, and moral and civilisational superiority, of the white settler population. WP, a married settler woman described in police notes as 'respectable and quiet', complained that she was raped by an African man on 27 February 1928, while returning home from a walk with a female friend. Two medical practitioners, Dr Kauntze of Laboratory Services and Dr MacKinnon, a doctor practising at Nairobi, testified in the case. MacKinnon examined WP on the evening of the assault and found that she was suffering from shock, swollen eyes, and bruising to her face, neck and shoulders. He could find no genital injuries but explained—as for the cases described above—that evidence of penetration would not be expected in a married woman, and so the lack of injury was 'consistent with penetration having taken place'. Accounting for the lack of spermatozoa found in WP's vagina, he suggested that 'in the struggle' the assailant had ejaculated outside her body. Kauntze argued that as the accused was suffering from gonorrhoea, his penis was possibly so inflamed that sperm could not pass through it. Demonstrating the contested nature of medical evidence (Ruberg 2013), and the meanings attached to it, the doctors disagreed as to other bodily signs of rape. Whereas MacKinnon argued that he did not consider bruising of the thighs would be present necessarily, Kauntze disagreed. In his view, bruising would be present if the woman had shown 'strong resistance'. As a corollary, he suggested that the psychiatric impact of assault might account for the absence of expected injuries, arguing that 'in some temperament there would be such mental disturbance as to cause little resistance'. Kauntze and MacKinnon, while differing in their views as to expected bodily and forensic indicators of rape, nevertheless concurred that violence was likely to have occurred and offered explanations for why expected evidence might not be present. WP was thus constructed in the medical evidence in contradictory ways, as both strongly resisting and helplessly submitting to her assailant through terror. Referencing the medical evidence in his judgement, Mr Justice Barth accepted that it would be unusual to find evidence of even forced intercourse in a married woman, and that she had been 'reduced to a more or less helpless condition' by the assault. Finding that there was 'no room for doubt' as to the veracity of WP's story, he sentenced her assailant to death, making this the first case where capital punishment was imposed since the law was amended in 1926 (KNA AC/1/338; *East African Standard* 28 April 1928; 20 July 1928).

Such ideas of white women's respectability and virtue persisted throughout the colonial period. In the 1949 case of GMS described earlier, MO Littlejohn, testified to finding bruising and scratches to her thighs and arms. He noted that there was 'no external evidence of damage' except a 'small linear split' near the vaginal entrance. Suggesting that penetration was a possible cause for the split, Littlejohn nonetheless posited that he would not expect to find genital injury in a woman who 'had been married'. As in WP's case described above, the judge drew upon notions of respectability to contextualise the medical evidence and suggested that even if medical evidence was lacking, the case was clearly rape. Mr. Justice Thacker noted that the corroboration required in rape cases was not fixed, but 'varies in different circumstances'. He informed assessors that 'the word of a prostitute' would require 'very grave corroboration indeed' but in GMS's case, as a 'virtuous elderly European woman...I do not consider that much corroboration is required' and that it would be sufficient to convict if only 'slight...or partial' penetration had been proved. Reminding assessors of the racial dimensions of the case, he stated that 'it is scarcely necessary to point out to you that if she was raped by these two Africans, there certainly never was any question of her consenting to it'. Both men were sentenced to death (AXM1/8/367).[2]

As Elizabeth Thornberry (2019) has found for South Africa, however, not all European women benefited from presumptions of respectability and credibility. Those suspected of transgressing racial boundaries or behaving in sexually immoral ways were at risk of having their cases undermined, reflecting contemporaneous concerns with white women's sexuality (Jackson 2013). Medical evidence could be interpreted in such circumstances to cast doubt on the woman's story. MF, a thirty-eight-year-old European woman living at Eldoret complained of having been raped by a Nandi man as she walked home from a friend's house on 22 January 1928. Medical examination found that 'penetration had been effected in a legal sense'. No seminal discharge was found on the complainant's clothes, perhaps because they had been washed before police seized them. It is clear from the correspondence that police and prosecuting authorities had misgivings about the case. Mr. Wolseley-Bourne, Acting Deputy Commissioner of Police, alerted colleagues that he had 'heard various theories regarding this case—all of a very confidential nature', while the committing magistrate Mr Wightman recorded that he 'must confess difficulty in reconciling the description of the assault as given by the complainant with the medical evidence', a statement which the Solicitor-General, Mr. McCarthy, stated he was 'at a loss to understand', as the reasons for this assertion were omitted from the record of the committal proceedings. Eldoret Police Superintendent Captain Rainsford wrote to McCarthy to explain that, in his opinion, the complainant 'is not telling the whole truth...She has a reputation of being a "Teaser" and...she would be able to show bruises on her body any day after she had been horse-playing with male friends, as is her habit'. Rainsford drew on medical evidence to underline his point, stating that 'the injuries found were not as severe as one would expect if she had a struggle with a buck native'. Rainsford suggested that she had been 'playing the fool' with a European male friend she had visited before the assault, and on her way home she met the accused, 'gave him a certain amount of encouragement', and then 'got frightened, struggled, and reported the matter'

[2] See also the 1945 case of attempted rape on two European girls, where Crown Counsel contacted the MO in the case, asking him if he could push his medical evidence further to prove 'even the slightest penetration' which would have resulted in a charge of rape (KNA AXM1/8/112).

(KNA AG/52/391). MF's alleged actions, in a period of high anxiety about so-called 'Black Peril' and the vulnerability of white women to assault by African men (Anderson 2010), were thus constructed as transgressive. If Rainsford was correct, she had not only breached social and sexual boundaries, but also potentially the law, as a white woman 'enticing or soliciting' an African man to have intercourse was a misdemeanour punishable by up to two years' imprisonment (Barth et al. 1924, 734). The Supreme Court transcripts for this case do not survive in the file, so it is difficult to trace how these questions played out in court, but ultimately Mr. Justice Barth declared the case 'extremely weak' and acquitted the accused (*East African Standard*, 17 April 1928). This case demonstrates how, in cases where a European woman's respectability and conformity to racial boundaries were questioned, medical evidence could be used to undermine rather than to bolster her allegations. Thus, interracial sexual violence cases did not straightforwardly follow the logics of 'Black Peril' (Thornberry 2019, 10).

Medico-legal evidence also highlights the racialised operation of colonial justice around views on emotional impacts of sexual violence on European versus African women. Only one case in the dataset here involving African complainants involved medical testimony on the emotional state of a victim. Examining NN on 7 September 1947 after she had been raped by a group of 20 men in Nairobi, Dr. Singh, Sub-Assistant Surgeon at Nairobi General Dispensary, noted that she 'was nervous' when he examined her and 'was disturbed about what had happened', a state that was perhaps exacerbated by the fact that she had been examined at the same time as one of her assailants (KNA AC/2/637). As Joanna Bourke (2012) and Pauline Dirven (2024) note, psychological and emotional harms of sexual violence were marginalised by the medical community until the late 1950s, and did not become widely discussed until the 1970s, reflecting the impact of second-wave feminist theories. However, in Kenya, the potential emotional harm of sexual violence was recognised for European women, particularly in cases where the alleged assailant was African, demonstrating that medical responses to sexual harms were racialised. This can be seen in the so-called 'Kijabe outrage' case of 1926, which led to the amendment of the law to make rape a capital crime in Kenya. JU, a 69-year-old European woman, was raped by two African men on 17 May 1926 (KNA AG/52/393). One of the examining doctors, Nakuru District Surgeon Henderson testified that '[JU] will never recover from the shock' (*East African Standard* 21 June 1926). The potential emotional impact on JU was reflected in her exceptional treatment elsewhere in the colonial legal system. At the committal hearing, JU was allowed to give evidence while holding her son's hand, and was provided with extra cushions as she gave her testimony (Ibid), while at the Supreme Court the Solicitor-General, Mr. Bown, asked that her son be allowed to sit next to her as she testified (*East African Standard* 4 August 1926).[3]

More than twenty years later, in the 1949 case of GMS described above, Dr. Littlejohn, MO, examined GMS and provided meticulous details of her injuries. He testified that upon examination 'she was distressed and shocked. Her pulse rate was 112 per minute', which he stated could be in keeping with her 'mental distress' (KNA AXM1/8/367). In recognition of the potential emotional impact of the assault and trial, GMS was questioned very delicately by counsel. Mr. Parry for the defence, asked her if she may have misidentified her assailant on account of being 'overwrought' due to emotional distress and fear (KNA AXM1/8/367). Potential emotional or psychological harms, then, were recognised for European women, but not usually for African women and girls. The lack of attention to African women's potential emotional suffering reflected prevalent attitudes which are neatly summarised in the views attributed to Mr. Justice Connell in 1956, that 'in many cases of rape the offence is not a serious one, particularly African-African cases' (KNA AP/1/1845), in contrast with African courts which treated rape as a serious offence (Shadle 2008). It could also be seen as a reflection of colonial psychiatric discourses—strongly influenced by scientific racism, discriminatory ethnopsychiatry, and notions of cultural relativity influenced by colonial anthropology—which posited that Africans did not have the complex inner lives afforded to Europeans (Shadle 2017; McCulloch 1995). Yet, despite the failure of colonial medical officials to recognise the emotional harms of sexual assault, African women and their witnesses testified powerfully to the emotional as well as physical pain caused by such violence, demonstrating how women used the court setting to contest colonial narratives (Schmidt 1990; Roberts 2005). RS complained that she had been raped in the forest near Kabete in January 1945. Medical evidence taken at the General Dispensary at Nairobi disclosed injuries to her knee and hand but did not indicate her emotional state. In her testimony, RS emphasised her fear and distress as she attempted

[3] For other cases where the emotional impact on European complainants is acknowledged, see KNA AC/1/338; KNA AM/1/5.

to escape the accused, stating 'I was just running away blindly…I did not know what was the accused's mind and I did not know then what he wanted to do to me. I was frightened'. Testifying in support of her complaint, her husband articulated that she was 'very sorrowful' when he first saw her after the assault (KNA AC/2/501). Thus, African women, and their witnesses, claimed their emotional distress, despite the colonial medico-legal system's denial of that impact.

## 5 Conclusion

Medico-legal responses to sexual violence in present-day Kenya remain under-resourced and beset by challenges relating to economic inequalities and disparities in access to healthcare facilities. Yet, these are not new issues, but rather are colonial legacies. Through examining sexual violence cases in colonial Kenya, this chapter has historicised these concerns, demonstrating that survivors and victims of violence in the past experienced similar obstacles to medical care. It is contended that these obstacles were rooted in the colonial logics of a racially-stratified settler society. Spatial segregation, the prioritisation of funding for European healthcare facilities at the expense of African communities, the development of key infrastructure such as roads around the needs of settlers, contributed to difficulties and delays in accessing care, which were compounded by racist ideas about the seriousness of sexual violence against African women and girls, and sometimes by poor handling of forensic evidence. This contrasted strongly with the comparatively quick and thorough care that European women and girls, often sharing the same social milieu as medical officers, received.

As well as the practical implications of settler colonial policies for African women and girls experiencing sexual violence, the racialised and gendered operation of colonial law inflected the uses and meanings of medical evidence in sexual violence cases. Given the primacy placed on chronological age by sexual offence laws, medical expertise was used to determine the age of complainants, privileging markers of physiological development over local conceptions of age as a social category contingent, for example, on whether a girl had been initiated according to local custom. Medical evidence could also be used as proof—or otherwise—of a woman's complaint, but the meanings of similar evidence were interpreted differently according to the racialised position of women within colonial Kenyan society, in ways which often benefited European women.

Bodily pain, and evidence of emotional distress, were, in general, more easily believed in cases where the victim was a European woman, especially where the alleged assailant was African. Yet, this was not a simple picture, and European women's claims of rape were not automatically believed. Notions of respectability impacted their credibility, with European women suspected of transgressing racial boundaries or behaving in sexually immoral ways likely to receive a less sympathetic hearing. Thus, in the final analysis, medico-legal evidence—and its producers—served to reproduce forms of knowledge which upheld and reinforced gendered and racialised categories and oppressions within the context of colonial Kenya.

**Acknowledgment** The author would like to acknowledge the invaluable research assistance of Alfred Anangwe, as well as the generosity of Stacey Hynd and Emma Yapp who offered insightful comments on earlier drafts.

**Funding** The research for this chapter was supported by the Wellcome Trust [Grant number: 205378/Z/16/Z], as part of the Sexual Harms and Medical Encounters (SHaME) project at Birkbeck, University of London.

## References

### Archival Sources

*Kenya National Archives, Nairobi, Kenya*
AC/1 series.
AC/2 series.
AG/52 series.
AM/1 series.
AP/1 series.
AXM1/8 series.
DC KSM/1 series.

### Primary Printed Sources

Story of Kijabe Case. *East African Standard,* 21 June 1926.
The Kijabe Outrage Case. *East African Standard,* 4 August 1926.
Child Welfare. *The Democrat,* 21 January 1928.
Verdict in the Soy Assault Case. *East African Standard,* 17 April 1928.

Extreme Penalty Imposed in the Nairobi Assault Case. *East African Standard*, 28 April 1928.

Two Executions. *East African Standard*, 20 July 1928.

Woman Missionary Murdered. *East African Standard*, 6 January 1930.

Rape Appeal Dismissed. *East African Standard*, 2 February 1946.

Barth, J., R. Lyall Grant, H. Brown, and B. Crean eds. 1926. *The Laws of Kenya, Containing the Ordinances of Kenya in Force on the 1st Day of January, 1924*. Nairobi: Government Printer.

Government and Colony of Kenya. 1927. *Judicial Department Annual Report 1925*. Nairobi: Government Printer.

Government and Colony of Kenya. 1931. *Judicial Department Annual Report 1930*. Nairobi: Government Printer.

Kingdon, Donald. 1948. *The Laws of Kenya in Force on the 21st Day of September, 1948*. Nairobi: Government Printer.

## Secondary Sources

Ajema, C., W. Mukoma, N. Kilonzo, B. Bwire, and K. Otwombe. 2011. Challenges Experienced by Service Providers in the Delivery of Medico-Legal Services to Survivors of Sexual Violence in Kenya. *Journal of Forensic and Legal Medicine* 18: 162–166.

Anderson, David M. 2010. Sexual Threat and Settler Society: Black Perils in Kenya, c.1907–1930.*Journal of Imperial and Commonwealth History* 38: 47–74.

Bates, Victoria. 2016. *Sexual Forensics in Victorian and Edwardian England: Age, Crime, and Consent in the Court*. Basingstoke: Palgrave Macmillan.

Beck, Ann. 1981. *Medicine, Tradition and Development in Kenya and Tanzania, 1920–1970*. Waltham, MA: Crossroads Press.

Benson, Koni, and Joyce M. Chadya. 2005. *Ukubhinya:* Gender and Sexual Violence in Bulawayo, Colonial Zimbabwe, 1946–1956. *Journal of Southern African Studies* 31: 587–610.

Bernault, Florence. 2007. The Shadow of Rule: Colonial Power and Modern Punishment in Africa. In *Cultures of Confinement: A History of the Prison in Africa, Asia, and Latin America*, ed. Frank Dikötter and Ian Brown, 55–94. Ithaca: Cornell University Press.

Bridger, Emily, and Erin Hazan. 2022. Surfeit and Silence: Sexual Violence in the Apartheid Archive. *African Studies* 83: 286–305.

Chirwa, Danwood M. 2016. Access to Medicines and Health Care in Sub-Saharan Africa: A Historical Perspective. *Maryland Journal of International Law* 31: 21–43.

Cooper, Barbara. 1997. *Marriage in Maradi: Gender and Culture in a Hausa Society in Niger, 1900–1989*. Portsmouth: Heinemann.

Crozier, Anna. 2007. *Practising Colonial Medicine: The Colonial Medical Service in British East Africa*. London: I. B. Tauris.
Decker, Corrie. 2021. Sexuality in Colonial Africa: Current Trends and New Directions. In *Routledge Companion to Sexuality and Colonialism*, ed. Chelsea Schields and Dagmar Herzog, 42–54. Abingdon: Routledge.
Dirven, Pauline. 2024. Detached from Sympathy, Unconscious of Trauma: The Impact of the Forensic Virtues of Impartiality and Detachment on Rape Examinations in Britain 1924–1978. *Social History of Medicine*. https://doi.org/10.1093/shm/hkad097.
Du Mont, J., and D. Parnis. 2000. Sexual Assault and Legal Resolution: Querying the Medical Collection of Forensic Evidence. *Medicine and Law* 19: 779–792.
Fuentes, Marisa. 2016. *Disposessed Lives: Enslaved Women, Violence, and the Archive*. Philadelphia: University of Pennsylvania Press.
Grier, Beverly. 2004. Child Labour and Africanist Scholarship: A Critical Overview. *African Studies Review* 47: 1–25.
Hale, Matthew. 1736–1739. *Historia Placitorum Coronae: The History of the Pleas of the Crown*, vol. 1. London: Sollom Emlyn.
Hammonds, Evelyn M. 1997. Toward a Genealogy of Black Female Sexuality: The Problematic of Silence. In *Feminist Theory and the Body: A Reader*, ed. Janet Price and Margrit Shildrick, 249–259. New York: Taylor and Francis.
Human Rights Watch. 2021. *'I Had Nowhere to Go': Violence Against Women and Girls During the Covid-19 Pandemic in Kenya*. New York: Human Rights Watch.
Ilinca, Stefania, Laura Di Giorgio, Paola Salari and Jane. Chuma. 2019. Socio-Economic Inequality and Inequity in Use of Health Care Services in Kenya: Evidence from the Fourth Kenya Household Health Expenditure and Utilization Survey. *International Journal for Equity in Health* 18: 1–13.
Jackson, Will. 2017. *Madness and Marginality: The Lives of Kenya's White Insane*. Manchester: Manchester University Press.
Jackson, Will. 2013. Dangers to the Colony: Loose Women and the "Poor White" Problem in Kenya. *Journal of Colonialism and Colonial History* 14. https://doi.org/10.1353/cch.2013.0029
Jentzen, Jeffrey. 2019. Death and Empire: Medicolegal Investigations and Practice Across the British Empire. In *Global Forensic Cultures: Making Fact and Justice in the Modern Era*, ed. Ian A. Burney and Christopher Hamlin, 149–173. Baltimore: Johns Hopkins University Press.
Kennedy, Dane. 1987. *Islands of White: Settler Society and Culture in Kenya and Southern Rhodesia, 1890–1939*. Durham, NC: Duke University Press.
Keyse, Rhian Elinor. 2019. Imperial, International, and Local Responses to Early and Forced Marriage in British Colonial Africa, c.1920–1962. Unpublished PhD Thesis, University of Exeter.
Kilonzo, N., S. J. Theobald, E. Nyamato, C. Ajema, H. Muchela, J. Kibaru, E. Rogena, and M. Taegtmeyer. 2009a. Delivering Post-Rape Care Services:

Kenya's Experience in Developing Integrated Services. *Bulletin of the World Health Organization* 87: 555–559.

Kilonzo, N., N. Ndung'u, N. Nthamburi, C. Ajema, M. Taegtmeyer, S. Theobald, and R. Tolhurst. 2009b. Sexual Violence Legislation in Sub-Saharan Africa: The Need for Strengthened Medico-Legal Linkages. *Reproductive Health Matters* 17: 10–19.

Kolsky, Elizabeth. 2010. 'The Body Evidencing the Crime': Rape on Trial in Colonial India, 1860–1947. *Gender and History* 22: 109–130.

Landau, Paul. 1996. Explaining Surgical Evangelism in Colonial Southern Africa: Teeth, Pain and Faith. *Journal of African History* 37: 261–281.

Lee, Rebekah. 2021. *Health, Healing, and Illness in African History*. New York: Bloomsbury.

Mamdani, Mahmood. 1996. *Citizen and Subject: Contemporary Africa and the Legacy of Late Colonialism*. Princeton: Princeton University Press.

McCulloch, Jock. 1995. *Colonial Psychiatry and the African Mind*. Cambridge: Cambridge University Press.

Mertens, Charlotte. 2023. In the Ruins of Empire: Historicizing Sexual Violence in Congo. *International Feminist Journal of Politics* 25: 529–550.

Middleton, John, and Greet Kershaw. 1965. *The Kikuyu and Kamba of Kenya*. London: International African Institute.

Muinde, Jacinta, and Ruth Prince. 2023. A New Universalism? Universal Health Coverage and Debates About Rights, Solidarity, and Inequality in Kenya. *Social Science and Medicine* 319: 1–9.

Mulla, Sameena. 2014. *The Violence of Care: Rape Victims, Forensic Nurses, and Sexual Assault Intervention*. New York: New York University Press.

National Crime Research Centre. 2015.*Gender Based Violence in Kenya*. Nairobi: National Crime Research Centre.

Ndege, George. 2002. *Health, State, and Society in Kenya: Faces of Contact and Change*. Rochester, NY: Boydell and Brewer.

Ngutuku, Elizabeth, and Auma Okwany. 2024. Beyond Colonial Politics of Identity: Being and Becoming Female Youth in Colonial Kenya. *Genealogy* 8: 1–24.

Ochieng', William R. 1988. Colonial Famines in Luoland, Kenya, 1905–1945. *Transafrican Journal of History* 17: 21–33.

Odinga, Agnes. 2001. Women's Medicine and Fertility: A Social History of Reproduction in South Nyanza, Kenya, 1920–1980. Unpublished PhD thesis, University of Minnesota.

Olson, Rose, Wendy Macias-Konstantopoulos, Roseline Muchai, Katy Johnson, Ranit Mishori, and Brett Nelson. 2022. Development and Validation of a Data Quality Index for Forensic Documentation of Sexual and Gender-Based Violence in Kenya. *PLoS ONE*. https://doi.org/10.1371/journal.pone.0262297.

Ombongi, K., M. Dobson, M. Malowany, and R. Snow. 1998. The East African Medical Journal: Its History and Contribution to Regional Malaria Research During the Last 75 Years. *East African Medical Journal* 75: S10–S19.

Ominde, Simeon. 1952. *The Luo Girl: From Infancy to Marriage*. London: Macmillan.

Overton, John. 1987. The Colonial State and Spatial Differentiation: Kenya, 1895–1920. *Journal of Historical Geography* 13: 267–282.

Park, Emma. 2014. The Routes of Rule: The Role of Roads in Kenyan Governance and Popular Evaluations of 'Development' and Authority, 1890s–1992. Unpublished MA Thesis, Concordia University.

Quinlan, Andrea. 2017. *The Technoscientific Witness of Rape: Contentious Histories of Law, Feminism, and Forensic Science*. Toronto: University of Toronto Press.

Ranger, Terence. 1993. The Invention of Tradition Revisited: The Case of Colonial Africa. In *Legitimacy and the State in Twentieth Century Africa*, ed. Terence Ranger and Olufemi Vaughan, 62–111. London: Palgrave Macmillan.

Reuther, Jessica. 2018. Irresponsible Boys, Promiscuous Girls: Maturity, Gender, and Rape Myths in the Criminal Tribunals of Colonial Dahomey, 1924–1940. *Revue d'histoire de l'enfance « irrégulière »* 20: 67–84.

Roberts, Richard. 2005. *Litigants and Households: African Disputes and Colonial Courts in the French Soudan, 1896–1912*. Portsmouth, NH: Heinemann.

Rockowitz, Sarah, James Rockey, Laura Stevens, Melissa Colloff, Wangu Kanja, and Heather Flowe. 2023. Evaluating Case Attrition Along the Medico-Legal Case Referral Pathway for Sexual and Domestic Violence Survivors in Kenya: A Secondary Data Analysis. *Victims and Offenders* 19: 1104–1127.

Ruberg, Willemijn. 2013. Trauma, Body, and Mind: Forensic Medicine in Nineteenth-Century Dutch Rape Cases. *Journal of the History of Sexuality* 22: 85–104.

Schmidt, Elizabeth. 1990. Negotiated Spaces and Contested Terrain: Men, Women, and the Law in Colonial Zimbabwe, 1890–1939. *Journal of Southern African Studies* 16: 622–648.

Scully, Pamela. 1995. Rape, Race, and Colonial Culture: The Sexual Politics of Identity in the Nineteenth-Century Cape Colony, South Africa. *American Historical Review* 100: 335–359.

Shadle, Brett. 2008. Rape in the Courts of Gusiiland, Kenya, 1940s–1960s. *African Studies Review* 51: 27–50.

Shadle, Brett. 2017. *The Souls of White Folk: White Settlers in Kenya, 1900s–1920s*. Manchester: Manchester University Press.

Singh, Gagan Preet. 2021. Forensics, Body and State Power in South Asia: Recent Interventions and Their Importance. *History Compass* 19. https://doi.org/10.1111/hic3.12693.

Southall, Aidan. 1952. *Lineage Formation Among the Luo*. London: Oxford University Press.

Sowemimo, Annabel. 2023. *Divided: Racism, Medicine, and Why We Need to Decolonise Healthcare*. London: Profile.
Temmerman, Marleen, Emilomo Ogbe, Griffins Manguro, Iqbal Khandwalla, Mary Thiongo, Kishor Mandaliya, Lou Dierick, Markus MacGill, and Peter Gichangi. 2019. The Gender-Based Violence and Recovery Centre at Coast Provincial General Hospital, Mombasa, Kenya: An Integrated Care Model for Survivors of Sexual Violence. *PLoS Medicine* 16. https://doi.org/10.1371/journal.pmed.1002886
Thomas, Lynn. 2003. *Politics of the Womb: Women, Reproduction, and the State in Kenya*. Berkeley: University of California Press.
Thornberry, Elizabeth. 2019. *Colonizing Consent: Rape and Governance in South Africa's Eastern Cape*. Cambridge: Cambridge University Press.
Vaughan, Megan. 1991. *Curing Their Ills: Colonial Power and African Illness*. Cambridge: Polity Press.
Wagner, Günter. 1949. *The Bantu of North Kavirondo*, vol. 1. London: Oxford University Press.
Walters, Sarah. 2016. 'Child! Now You Are': Identity Registration, Labour, and the Definition of Childhood in Colonial Tanganyika, 1910–1950. *Journal of the History of Childhood and Youth* 9: 66–86.
Wangamati, Cynthia, Johanne Sundby, Chimaraoke Izugbara, Erick Nyambedha, and Ruth Prince. 2021. Challenges in Supporting Survivors of Child Sexual Abuse in Kenya: A Qualitative Study of Government and Non-Governmental Organizations. *Journal of Interpersonal Violence* 36. https://doi.org.https://doi.org/10.1177/0886260519846864.
White, Luise. 1990. *The Comforts of Home: Prostitution in Colonial Nairobi*. Chicago: Chicago University Press.
Williams, Elizabeth. 2018. 'Stoop Low to Conquer': Race and Sexual Trusteeship in the Kenyan 'Indian Crisis' of 1923. *Journal of Colonialism and Colonial History* 19. https://doi.org/10.1353/cch.2018.0021.
Wright, Stephanie. 2023. 'Facts That Are Declared Proven': Sexual Violence, Forensic Medicine, and the Courtroom in Early Francoist Spain. *Women's History Review* 32: 939–959.

# A Crisis of Consent? Police Surgeons, Rape and HIV/AIDS in Late Twentieth-Century Britain

*George J. Severs*

## 1 Introduction

Around the spring of 1986, John Campbell was arrested. Suspected of dealing drugs and pimping out younger boys, Campbell was in fact a fellow sex worker who had been caught with a personal supply of Class A drugs. Despite being only eighteen years old at the time, Campbell had been a sex worker for several years in and around Piccadilly Circus, known to its rent boys, their clients and the police as 'the Dilly' (Reed 2013). His protective guidance to other 'Dilly boys' had been misconstrued as pimping, just one example in a long history of the criminalisation of care within sex work (Slagstad and Kveim 2022; Laite 2012). According to Campbell, having been arrested he was 'held in the wing overnight, medical the next day, told I had to have an HIV test—and I said I've already had one. And they said well that doesn't mean that you're not positive now, so you have to have another test'. With little choice, Campbell made his preferences clear: he did not want to be 'in an isolation

G. J. Severs (✉)
Geneva Graduate Institute, Geneva, Switzerland
e-mail: george.severs@graduateinstitute.ch



R. E. Keyse et al. (eds.), *Sexual Violence in Medicine and Psychiatry*, Genders and Sexualities in History,
https://doi.org/10.1007/978-3-032-10800-5_11

room like the last one'—his previous arrests seem to have resulted in similar experiences. This time was different: 'they said, no, this time you'll go onto the actual hospital wing, you'll be in a cell on your own but you'll go onto the actual hospital wing'. It was on the hospital wing that Campbell received his HIV diagnosis: 'The doctor came back in and said "Mr Campbell, you had an HIV test last time you were here". And I said "yeah". He said, "the results were positive"' (John Campbell interview).

Campbell's diagnosis experience is revealing on several fronts, but two aspects stand out: that his HIV diagnosis was occasioned by his interaction with the criminal legal system, and that he was forced to undergo an HIV test. The medical and juridical structures which scaffolded this experience collided to remove Campbell's ability to consent to medical testing. Contemporary biomedical ethics emphasise the need for informed consent as part of a medical procedure, particularly those which involve 'giving a biological specimen' such as a blood or tissue sample (Lee et al. 2019: 110). This was also the prevailing view amongst medical researchers across the period this chapter discusses, but during these years the primacy of informed consent was less stable, largely (but not exclusively) due to AIDS-related concerns (Gillon 1987; Cancer Research Campaign Working Party in Breast Conservation 1983; Tobias and Souhami 1993). In the coercive environment of the 'medical wing'—presumably of HMP Chelmsford where Campbell was on remand—his option to consent was removed.

This chapter explores the ways in which medical doctors who worked with the police and victims of crime dealt with the emergence of the HIV test, the questions about consent which it engendered, and the ways in which rape and sexual violence cases shaped HIV testing practice. Debates in the wider medical research literature ran parallel to those in journals aimed at doctors who worked within the criminal legal system (Gillon 1987). This chapter focuses predominantly on the latter, mostly on 'police surgeons', precisely because they reveal the centrality of rape and sexual assault cases in the creation of implicit policies around testing. The post of police surgeon was created by the 1829 Metropolitan Police Act. As Joanna Bourke, one of the few historians to have worked on police surgeons explains, 'Any person with a medical degree could be appointed to the role, but the majority were GPs' (General Practitioners) working part-time except in major cities where higher crime rates demanded full time roles (Bourke 2018,713). By the mid-1980s, being a police surgeon was a more professionalised, full-time medical role, albeit one with unattractive hours and remuneration (Ibid 717). In 1994, the Association of Police Surgeons changed its name to the Association of Forensic Physicians as part of a broader organisational recentring of medicine (and decentring of police work).

What police surgeons thought about their patients' consent to HIV testing matters to historians of sexual violence not only because it reveals how a portion of the medical profession thought about consent, confidentiality and bodily autonomy. It also matters because police surgeons were likely to be involved in the testing and treating of those involved in sexual assault and rape cases, both as victims and perpetrators (Bourke 2018; Dirven 2024). Understanding how police surgeons conceptualised and practised consent during HIV testing helps us to reconstruct the experiences of victim/survivors more fully, and demonstrates the impact of sexual violence in shaping HIV testing policy in the late 1980s.[1] Recent work on the ways in which medicine has been manipulated by reactionary or abusive forces draws attention to the ways in which consent did, or did not, feature in working practices (Rusterholz and Kelly 2025; Thomlinson 2016, 168). Understanding the way consent played into policies which were formulated in response to new medical developments, such as the HIV test, forms part of the broader corpus of consent, power, and bioethics which sexual violence scholarship inhabits. It also contributes to scholarship on HIV/AIDS within criminal legal frameworks which have rightly identified carceral settings as inhibiting patient/prisoner access to healthcare, including HIV testing (Day 2023). As this chapter makes clear, HIV testing could be used coercively and illiberally at the intersection of medical and criminal legal settings.

This chapter focuses on police surgeons and forensic medics working in Great Britain, but especially the jurisdiction of England and Wales. The professional association of police surgeons covered 'Great Britain' (despite having members in Northern Ireland), but physicians from England dominated its proceedings. Moreover, despite Edinburgh's reputation as the 'AIDS capital of Europe' because of the high proportion of intravenous (IV) drug use there (Elizabeth 2022, 168–169), it was the jurisdiction of England and Wales in which the highest numbers of HIV/AIDS cases were seen during the period, as well as being where most of

[1] Throughout this chapter I refer to both 'victims' and 'survivors' of sexual violence. I discuss the deployment of these terms in Severs (2024b).

the police surgeons engaged in published discussions about HIV/AIDS, consent and sexual violence were based.

The historical literature on police surgeons is small, though a few historians have given serious consideration to the ways in which police surgeons engaged with victims of rape and sexual assault (Bourke 2018; Dirven 2024). Bourke has suggested that police surgeons ricocheted between 'cultures of harm and care' from the 1960s, cultures which played out clearly in their uneven practices of caring for rape victims (Bourke 2018). This chapter further explores the ways in which police surgeons managed this uneasy balance, stemming from their sometimes competing demands as workers within medical and criminal legal systems. In doing so, it contributes to ongoing critiques of the term 'criminal justice system', identifying coercive medical practices within what was in fact a series of interconnected juridical *systems* which many identified as unjust (Levin 2023). The ways in which police surgeons responded to the HIV test, particularly the place of patient consent to such testing, reveals that an ethos of care prevailed in the late twentieth century alongside the potential for coercion. As I will demonstrate, there was a crisis of consent in the mid-1980s. Recognising this serves as a useful reminder of the fragility of the right of patients to consent when periods of national, particularly medical, emergencies are marshalled to trump the rights of vulnerable or minoritised individuals. This crisis of consent was short-lived, and otherwise the place of consent in the history of police surgeon thinking around HIV testing is one of broad continuity. In exploring this, it is possible to see an aspect of what the historian Virginia Berridge has identified as 'a particular form of liberal consensus round AIDS' in Britain taking shape, and doing so in often illiberal criminal legal settings (Berridge 1996, 55). Doing so further highlights the unbalanced power dynamics at play between doctors and patients. Histories of HIV/AIDS have emphasised the rise of the 'patient expert' (Ware 2019, 117–120), but we would do well to remember that this shift occurred alongside the continuation of patient groups with minimal power over their care or bodily autonomy. I therefore refer, where appropriate, to the 'patient/prisoner' to highlight the carceral and potentially coercive environments in which these HIV histories played out.

## 2 First Impressions: HIV/AIDS and Testing in the Mid-1980s

As a result of work by virologists at the Middlesex Hospital and scientists at the Chester Beatty Institute (now the Institute for Cancer Research), a test for HIV became 'widely available' around October 1985 (Berridge 1996, 46, 51–2 and 92). One month later, HIV/AIDS was mentioned for the first time in *The Police Surgeon*, the journal of the Association of Police Surgeons. This came in the form of a review of Derek Llewellyn-Jones' book *Herpes, AIDS and Other Sexually Transmitted Diseases.* It is likely that the emerging crisis around AIDS, rather than herpes, was of most interest to the journal, as few police surgeons considered sexual health as part of their remit. A survey of police surgeons carried out a year earlier had revealed that 'only 36 per cent prescribed medicine against sexually transmitted diseases' to women they dealt with following rape or sexual violence (Bourke 2018, 718). The review of Llewellyn-Jones' book reveals the kernel of interest in HIV/AIDS amongst police surgeons, and suggests some of their concerns about the virus as discussions about HIV testing were emerging. These concerns are particularly useful in reconstructing the landscape of anxieties around HIV/AIDS amongst police surgeons during the months in which HIV testing first became a possibility.

The unnamed reviewer recorded the 'terror and panic' of professionals dealing with HIV/AIDS. This was situated within a broader culture of anxieties around HIV/AIDS which accompanied the realisation that the virus was not confined to gay men, IV drug users or haemophiliacs, but had the potential to infect anyone (Cook 2017b). As the UK Government's public health television advert broadcast in 1987 informed its viewers, HIV/AIDS was 'now a danger that has become a threat to us all'. Police surgeons' panic preceded the national culture of unease in part because they understood the ways in which HIV was transmitted better than most. As qualified medics, most would have assimilated the knowledge that the virus was transmitted through bodily fluids (mostly semen and blood) which had been apparent for several years before the review of Llewellyn-Jones's book was published. Their concern, articulated by the anonymous reviewer, emerged from police surgeons' proximity to those most at risk of contracting HIV. The reviewer told his police surgeon readers that 'our police colleagues and their clients are involved so often with those most prone to harbour, nay to propagate, such serious ailments with their grave outlooks'. Here, the ailment was HIV and the 'grave outlook' was AIDS and, presumably, an AIDS-related death. The chances of such a 'grave' outcome was, the reviewer noted, 'minimal, yet the consequences may be dire' ('Book review' 1985, 79). The reviewer hoped that more information along the lines of Llewelyn-Jones' book would serve to allay some of the panic their colleagues were displaying, and welcomed its publication. They took issue, however, with the author's 'philosophy'. Llewellyn-Jones 'cannot be faulted for his desire to see patients "treated confidentially without any moral strictures being passed"' wrote the reviewer, 'but that does not excuse us from the need to have a stance ourselves. Where does emancipation stop and licence start?' (Ibid, 79–80). The reviewer was particularly concerned with 'greater promiscuity' which, they argued, 'must be the cause of the increased incidence of sexually transmitted diseases' (Ibid, 80).

Testing was not mentioned in this review, but the reviewer's underlying opposition to medical practice anchored in 'emancipation' points to early signs of the crisis of consent. Police surgeons like the reviewer were keen for more information about HIV/AIDS, but the nascent epidemic had ossified beliefs which were staunchly opposed to 'permissive' liberal attitudes towards sex (Cook 2017a). For the reviewer, sex was 'not simply a matter between two consenting adults... as police surgeons know only too well' and argued that there was a 'clear locus to express strong disapproval when attendance at genitourinary clinics has more than doubled in ten years' ('Book review' 1985, 80). These dual crises, of promiscuity and HIV/AIDS, led the reviewing police surgeon to question the sanctity of medical practices such as confidentiality and impartial treatment.

This early stance on HIV/AIDS did not set the tone for discussions of the virus within *The Police Surgeon*. A year later, in November 1986, James Hilton published an article on 'AIDS and the Police'. Hilton was by this point a long-serving and senior police surgeon. As Force Surgeon to the Norfolk Constabulary, he was the most senior police surgeon in the county, but Hilton's influence was national. Not only was he an elected member of the Council of the Association of Police Surgeons of Great Britain, he also co-edited *The New Police Surgeon*, a volume which informed the practice of many of his colleagues (Burges and Hilton 1978, 16–17). His, therefore, was an influential voice. Hilton's intervention addressed a culture of fear which continued to beset the police force, particularly amongst 'the beat officer' whom Hilton described (in gendered language which speaks to the male-dominated police service of

1980s Britain) as being 'naturally fearful for his own health and safety' because 'he knows [his duties] will bring him into contact inevitably with these very terrifying infections about which he knows little and understands less'. Hilton offered to 'point the way in which we should be advising our respective Chief Police Officers and, incidentally, how we should be looking after ourselves' (Hilton 1986, 120).

Unlike the review published the previous year, Hilton's article tackled the issue of testing for HIV. The merits of early HIV testing, particularly for police surgeons as a medical and prosecutorial tool in rape cases, had not yet been established (a development I discuss below). As a result, Hilton discussed HIV tests cautiously. 'Tests to determine whether a person has or has had the virus are not always accurate' he wrote, noting that they could 'take months to develop' and that 'several follow-up tests are always required' (Hilton 1986, 120–121). Hilton was not convinced of the short-term benefits of HIV testing but, in establishing a policy around testing patient/prisoners for HIV, his position was clear. 'ANY tests conducted on a person be he a suspected criminal or a police officer must be with his consent and the release of information about the result of the test must also be with that person's consent' (Hilton 1986, 122).

The capitalisation of the word 'ANY' in this emphatic directive suggests that Hilton was anticipating—or had experienced—the questioning of this approach, either from outright opposition or through conditions drawn from the juridical nature of the work. Hilton did attach some conditions, warning against acts of disclosure for reasons 'other than medical or public health'. For Hilton, reasons attached to policing or imprisonment did not trump the need for patient/prisoner consent in the way that, in incredibly rare circumstances, medical necessity might. As I have written about elsewhere, the late twentieth century saw debates over whether the consent of a person living with HIV was required for their HIV status to be disclosed by a third party. Some university staff, for example, objected to policies which demanded they never disclose the HIV status of their students, arguing that if an employer's reference asked for this they could be accused of providing false information (Severs 2024a, 118–120). Hilton's article, however, reveals the emphasis on consent by senior forensic medics in early discussions of HIV testing. Significantly, it also underscores that it was medical, rather than juridical arguments which had the potential to trump the insistence on consent. On the more authoritarian side of police surgeons' work, namely within the criminal legal system, consent was afforded primacy in HIV testing.

Hilton was not alone in emphasising the importance of consent and confidentiality in police surgeons' handling of HIV. A debate in the *British Medical Journal* in 1992 reveals that most police surgeons emphasised consent and confidentiality in their HIV-related work. The debate was sparked in response to a *BMJ* editorial written by Ken Mason, Emeritus Regius Professor of Forensic Medicine at the University of Edinburgh, on the recording of HIV status on police computers (Laurie 2017). Mason concluded that a balance needed to be struck (and, he argued, was being struck) between the need for police officers to know the HIV status of those in their charge and their prisoners' right to privacy, though he more heavily emphasised the former. The police, Mason suggested, were 'a particularly vulnerable group' who had 'a right to know if they had been or are being exposed to contagious disease' (Mason 1992, 995).

That Mason seemed to be suggesting that prisoners' rights to privacy were surpassed by police officers' need for 'protection' perturbed his colleagues. Letters from four forensic medical professionals were published in the *BMJ*, ranging from suggesting 'room for improvement' in an article which 'cries out for correction', to outright 'dismay...' ('Recording HIV status on police computers' 1992, 1243). Allison Jeynes, a physician who had researched HIV risk, pointed out that 'medical professional bodies insist on maintaining confidentiality and obtaining proper informed consent' before testing patients for HIV. A. J. Lyons, a London-based police surgeon, wrote that, despite being told by custody officers 'From time to time... "Doc, be careful, he's got HIV"', these warnings had never been validated. As such, Lyons could see 'no reason for the police to record this information at all'. Confidentiality and consent were principles which, for these police surgeons at least, were central to forensic HIV medicine.

To be sure, police surgeons' practice was not overtly liberal, even if Hilton's and those writing against Mason appeared to be. It was in the mid-1980s that, according to the historian Virginia Berridge, 'a particular form of liberal consensus' emerged in the UK, with testing for HIV acting as 'an important symbolic procedure in the establishment of a liberal policy line' (Berridge 1996, 55, 72). Carceral settings such as police stations and especially prisons, however, could not be described as liberal in either their operations or their responses to HIV/AIDS (though, as Janet Weston has pointed out, the response of prison authorities to HIV/

AIDS varied across Europe) (Weston 2022). Hilton's insistence on confidentiality and consent led him to 'the principle of treating any suspected case as if it were AIDS'. As he explained, 'In cases where a person in custody provides a sample which confirms AIDS and yet does not permit that information to be released, police officers could be at risk' (Hilton 1986, 122). Treating all suspected HIV/AIDS 'cases' 'as if it were AIDS', he argued, allowed workers within the criminal legal system to take adequate precautions without violating the need for the patient to consent to wide disclosure of their HIV status. This was in marked contrast to the ways in which other elements of the criminal legal system, notably prisons, were dealing with HIV testing, both in and beyond Britain. Weston's work on HIV/AIDS in prison contexts has revealed widespread concern that, in the UK, 'the confidentiality of test results was not respected within prisons' (Weston 2019, 228) and that, in countries including Ireland, 'Doctors shared the identities of those testing positive with prison management' (Weston 2022, 92; Day 2023). In both national contexts, such breaches in confidentiality led to policies of segregating HIV-positive prisoners on separate wings (Weston 2019, 228; Weston 2022, 92). Whilst police surgeons appeared to be more committed to their emphasis on consensual HIV testing, that commitment was not universal or inevitable.

## 3 Testing, Consent and Victims of Sexual Violence

That the primacy of consent was not guaranteed within police surgeons' practice reveals the ways in which a liberal testing policy could shield potentially coercive practices. For victims of rape and sexual abuse, whose refusal to consent had already been overridden, the potential for further coercion in medical or criminal legal settings was concerning. Police surgeons sat at the nexus of medical and criminal systems, one which victims of rape and sexual violence navigated. Conducting medical examinations of victims and perpetrators of various forms of sexual assault formed some eighteen per cent of police surgeons' workloads when these were surveyed in the mid-1960s, the third-highest element of their workload (Bourke 2018, 714). It is likely that this percentage increased in the late twentieth century, part of the 'rapid increase in reports of rape since the 1960s' (Bourke 2007, 15). Victims of rape were integral in establishing practices of HIV testing. Their cases demonstrated both the evidential importance of the HIV test *and* the need for those tests to be conducted consensually.

The number of rapes being dealt with by police surgeons was increasing at the same time as new ways of treating victims were being developed. The first Sexual Assault Referral Centre (SARC) was opened in 1986 in St Mary's Hospital, Manchester. Raine Roberts, a police surgeon who had been arguing for SARCs since the early 1980s, was appointed as its first Clinical Director. The numbers of women police surgeons was rising in this period, but slowly. The year before the St Mary's SARC was opened, a study found that there were over seven male police surgeons to every one of their female colleagues (Bourke 2018, 717). SARCs like St Marys offered dedicated spaces for victims of rape and sexual assault to undergo testing, treatment and therapy, an alternative to the 'cool detachment' with which police surgeons had treated rape victims until at least the early 1980s (Roberts 1987; Dirven 2024, 498). Police surgeons were not only responding to the new possibility of testing from the mid-1980s, but were increasingly doing so in new and particular sites specific to rape and sexual assault.

Roberts herself published articles which detailed her own experience of responding to new ways of testing for sexually transmitted infections. These articles illuminate changing attitudes of police surgeons towards sexual health testing and treatment, including for HIV. Roberts told her colleagues that she did 'not usually take swabs for gonorrhoea or other sexually transmitted diseases in rape victims'. The reason was not a lack of care or concern for such victims but rather, she argued, from concerns of a false negative test result. As she explained 'if the infection had been passed on during alleged rape only a few organisms might be present and might not be picked up on the swab. A negative result would give the woman a false sense of security'. In other words, testing for STIs was not standard practice amongst many police surgeons because, at the moment they were charged with examining victims, the chances of detecting them was low, leading to the risk of a false negative result. Instead, Roberts advised the victims of rape she examined 'to attend a Genito-Urinary Clinic in about a week's time' when the infection was more likely to be detectable (Roberts 1986, 31).

In 1986, then, testing rape victims for sexually transmitted infections was not standard practice for police surgeons, who tended not to see this as part of their medico-legal work. That year, though, a case with which Roberts was presented caused her to rethink her practice, and that of her fellow police surgeons. Roberts explained that 'A girl whom I saw a few weeks ago after she had complained of rape has now found that she has gonorrhoea'. Unsurprisingly, the added knowledge that her rape had led to a sexually transmitted infection had 'caused her extreme distress'. Adding to this distress was the fact that the alleged rapist in the case, whilst admitting he had gonorrhoea, was suggesting to police that he might have caught it from the victim. His allegation was that the victim's STI was evidence of her promiscuity 'and had consented to what occurred' (Roberts 1986, 31).

This case was instructive to Roberts. Having examined the victim shortly after the incident was reported, she had 'noted that the genital area was sore and red, the findings being consistent with her story'. However, in line with her usual practice (and that of most of her fellow police surgeons), Roberts had administered no tests for sexually transmitted infections. 'It would have been of great value', she conceded, 'to know whether gonorrhoea could have been found at the time of the examination'. If it had, the alleged rapist's version of events would have been more likely to have been believed. If no gonorrhoea was found, 'it would suggest that the infection had indeed been transmitted in the rape and had not become apparent until later'. Sexually transmitted infections, Roberts realised, were potential evidentiary links between presenting victims and their alleged rapists. Pushing back against the largely standard practice of not swabbing victims for such infections when they first presented to police surgeons, Roberts suggested that 'Perhaps we should think again' (Roberts 1986, 31).

That process of thinking again was not just undertaken by police surgeons. Other medical professionals, crucially those who dealt with victims of rape and sexual assault or abuse, were also grappling with HIV and the challenges which testing for the virus posed (not least as part of the evidentiary basis of proving the rape). Genitourinary medics, who diagnose and treat people with sexually transmitted infections, were also formulating ways in which to administer HIV tests during the 1980s. Unlike police surgeons, whose debates about HIV tests were always articulated broadly, genitourinary medics were particularly concerned about victims of sexual violence. Perhaps for this reason, the need for the patient's consent was not questioned. The policies and practices which hospital medics began to recommend reveal the ways in which the medical colleagues of police surgeons (who often collaborated with them on sexual assault cases) thought about testing for sexually transmitted infections. It points to a broader medical reckoning with HIV testing, particularly with the question of when they were useful, clinically and evidentially. Examining how genitourinary medics thought about HIV tests not only furthers our understanding of the ways in which medical professionals responded to the new possibility of such tests, it also reveals how doctors whose professional allegiance was clearly defined by medical rather than juridical practice engaged with questions posed by the criminal legal system when it came to consent, HIV and sexual violence.

One of the earliest reported cases came in 1987, when 'a 24-year-old woman was examined and tested for HIV' in St Mary's Hospital, London 'because she had been raped two weeks previously' (Murphy et al. 1989, 718). As is the case in the majority of rapes, the victim knew her rapist and, having forced her to have sex, he 'subsequently told her that he was positive for HIV'. Unlike in other cases, such as the one discussed above where victims subsequently discovered that they had contracted a sexually transmitted infection, here the victim had been told that her assailant was living with HIV, putting it on the agenda of her post-rape care immediately. This was becoming increasingly common during this period. A study of male rape victims published in 1991 found that over half had been threatened with HIV transmission by their assailants (Hillman et al. 1991, 22–24; Severs 2024b, 204). Using it as a tool to further inflict sexual violence, rapists were incidentally pushing HIV onto the genitourinary medical agenda.

Those who treated the victim at St. Mary's had a clear course of action: 'all adult victims of rape should be offered a test for HIV, reassured that the risk of infection is low, and offered counselling'. Their emphasis on HIV further indicates that it was the HIV/AIDS epidemic which prompted the turning point in how medics approached testing victims of rape and sexual assault. In addition to their medical role, though, juridical issues were also at play. Not only did they need to ascertain whether their patients were HIV positive, genitourinary medics were tasked with determining whether their positive patients had seroconverted as a result of their sexually violent encounter. In short, it was not just whether their patients who had been raped had HIV, but also whether their patients had HIV *because* they had been raped. Genitourinary medics may have been working squarely within the medical field, but they found themselves dealing with the same evidentiary questions as their police surgeon colleagues.

Despite the fact that it was police surgeons who sat uniquely at this intersection of medical and legal practice, discussing this important causative medical evidence was often left to genitourinary medics based in hospitals. In part, this may reflect the fact that police surgeons were beginning to transition away from their role 'within' the police service towards more medical roles. From the late-1970s, police surgeons began to talk of their work in terms of forensic medical examinations, and were increasingly identifying as Forensic Medical Examiners (FMEs). In relation to this shift, Bourke has argued that police surgeons were attempting 'to distance themselves from law enforcement agencies', highlighting their medical roles and decentring their place within the criminal legal system (Bourke 2018, 726). This was a significant shift from earlier in the twentieth century, when police surgeons 'aligned themselves more with the law than with medicine' (Bourke 2018, 718; Dirven 2024, 497). Nonetheless, it was hospital-based genitourinary medics who established a clear practice of HIV testing of rape victims. Writing in the *British Medical Journal*, the consultants at St Mary's in London who had examined the 24-year-old rape survivor offered their experience as an instructive example. When the woman initially visited the clinic in May 1987, she was tested for gonorrhoea, chlamydia and HIV. The results for all of these tests were negative but, because her rapist had 'told her that he was positive for HIV antibody' the clinicians tested her for HIV three months later, after which time they were confident that HIV would be detectable. Following this second test, doctors informed the woman that she was HIV-positive. Taken together (and alongside a clinical history which indicated no other sexual contact, drug use or blood transfusions in the months leading up to her rape) those results revealed that she had contracted HIV as a result of her rape.

This link was key. Three other women had previously attended St Mary's having survived acts of rape and were found to be HIV positive. Unlike with the woman who formed the basis of the St Mary's article, these women had not had samples taken from them and stored following their initial visit to the clinic. As a result, clinicians (and by extension the criminal legal system) could not prove that these women's rapists were the cause of their seroconversion to HIV. As the consultants from St Mary's put it 'HIV infection could not be definitely attributed to the assault' (Murphy et al. 1989, 718).

A simple but important suggestion emerged from this paper: if rape survivors were willing to be tested for HIV, then those tests should be taken as quickly as possible, despite the knowledge that HIV was unlikely to be visible in tests until three months after initial exposure. Those tests, and samples taken at that time, could be crucial evidence in proving whether a person's rapist had also transmitted HIV to their victim. Not only would this help rape survivors understand what had happened to them and allow clinicians to refer their patients for appropriate counselling, such practice was also potentially useful as a means of proving causality (that the rape led to HIV) in criminal legal settings. If it could be proven that a rapist had passed HIV to his victim, this was an exacerbating factor with the potential for a further charge of grievous bodily harm (though this would not occur until the early twenty-first century) (Dodds et al. 2009). With little formal advice, and the need to address both medical and criminal legal concerns, testing on first contact and three months later became a useful 'first step' in post-rape clinical practice, one which attracted international agreement soon after its publication (Foster and Bartlett 1989).[2]

The presence of HIV, and the challenges it posed in terms of its delayed presentation, was crucial in shaping the ways genitourinary medics dealt with victims of non-consensual sex, both medically and juridically. The consent of their patients to undergo such tests, however, appeared to be absolute. Let me return, though, to the question at the heart of this chapter: the emphasis on consent when testing people for HIV. It is clear that, for the genitourinary medics working at St. Mary's, their patients' consent was required in order to test for HIV. Yes, they impressed the medical and evidentiary value of not just one test but two, but the language they deployed in the *BMJ* indicates that this was a policy which operated consensually. Patients they encountered who had been raped 'should be *offered* a test for HIV' (emphasis added).

This had not always been the case. Beyond the work of police surgeons and genitourinary medics working with victims of rape, British physicians had been debating the 'need' for patient consent to undertake HIV tests. Mostly, these were confined to discussions of whether obtaining the consent of patients who had given blood samples for reasons other than HIV testing was necessary in research into the prevalence of HIV (Doll 1987; Gillon 1987). Such debates also took place between forensic medics

[2] Foster and Bartlett built on Murphy et al.'s contribution by arguing for the use of post exposure prophylaxes such as zidovudine.

who interacted with victims of rape and sexual abuse at the intersections of medical and criminal legal systems, including police surgeons.

## 4 Crisis of Consent

In the late 1980s, the emphasis on consent as part of HIV testing waivered. HIV/AIDS was now being spoken of as a 'crisis', heightening the emotionally charged responses to it. If police surgeons were embroiled in a culture of 'terror and panic' in 1985, as the *Police Surgeon* reviewer had noted that year, the United Kingdom more widely could be said to have caught up with them by 1987, which the historian Matt Cook identifies as the emotional epicentre of the epidemic (Cook 2017b). Indeed, Virginia Berridge characterises this period as one of 'wartime response' to the epidemic (Berridge 1996, 83–85). Historians have found utility in this bellicose metaphor in order to understand the urgency with which public health policy was created and to explain the hardening of public opinion against gay men in particular (Ibid; Cook 2017a). But perhaps there are other apt wartime comparisons to be made. Lawmakers have frequently used the sexual health of the armed services during or in anticipation of wartime as an excuse for passing coercive legislation which most often targeted sex workers (Cox 2007). If coercive policies designed to 'protect' the sexual health of the nation is a familiar feature of wartime, was the 'wartime response' to HIV/AIDS in Britain any different? As I now show, it was during this period of wartime response to AIDS that police surgeons waivered in their commitment to ensuring that tests and procedures relating to HIV were consensual. This departure from the insistence on consent was momentary and slight, but it reveals the cleavages in liberal consent policies which national emergencies and coercive carceral practices are able to exploit.

The April 1988 issue of *The Police Surgeon* sounded considerably more alarm at the ongoing HIV/AIDS epidemic than past issues had done. Three years had passed since audience members at the Association of Police Surgeon's annual general meeting had requested 'any advice on the subject of AIDS' ('Minutes' 1986, 16), with the lacuna of information heightening the growing sense of unease. The introduction to Selwyn Goldthorpe's article *AIDS and the Police Surgeon* was clear: given the alarming rise in the rates of infection, and the fact that the UK seemed to be just four years behind the numbers of cases being displayed in the USA (where infection rates were considerably higher), HIV/AIDS 'should affect the way all police surgeons work' (Goldthorpe 1988, 64).

Goldthorpe was, at the time, a police surgeon working in Liverpool, a city in the North West of England which, as I have discussed elsewhere, was reckoning with the 'arrival' of HIV/AIDS in its midst around the time Goldthorpe was writing (Severs 2024a, 21–23; Wetherell 2025, 306–315). His article ran through a pragmatic list of working practices which, he argued, would reduce the risk of HIV transmission from 'prisoner' to 'forensic examiner'. The crux of his argument was that, by identifying whether a 'prisoner' belonged to a category of person at highest risk of living with HIV, the police surgeon could change the ways they interacted with them to reduce their own risk of exposure to the virus. Goldthorpe identified nine 'high risk groups':

1. Prostitutes
2. Any drug addict that has shared a needle
3. Homosexuals
4. Haemophiliacs
5. Renal dialysis patients
6. The institutionalised, eg [sic.] prison
7. Tattooed
8. Multiple sexual partners
9. In contact with blood, eg [sic.] health workers, police (Goldthorpe 1988, 66).

Clearly, police surgeons were at routine risk of encountering members of these groups; physicians who recognised their own status as both healthcare professionals and part of the police service would have been justified in identifying themselves as a high-risk category in their own right. Generally, however, HIV/AIDS information articles, including this one, identified an external force (the prisoner) as the potential vector.

Goldthorpe concentrated most of his advice on work around needles. For many of his nine at-risk groups, needles were the most likely means of HIV entering the bloodstream, making this an unsurprising and pragmatic focus. He argued that there ought to be 'education of the police, who must be wary of searching addicts' pockets' because, for the police,

'Needle-stick injury is the commonest mode of transmission'.[3] Because of this, coupled with the fact that Goldthorpe had found half of addicts have 'used a needle at some stage', he argued that 'All addicts should be regarded as high risk'. To combat this risk, police officers and forensic examiners should 'get the prisoner to turn out his own pockets' before searching or examining them carefully because 'needles or syringes may be strapped to the inguinal area, or lumbar-sacral recess' (Goldthorpe 1988, 67).

Such practices were extensions of policies which predated the arrival of HIV/AIDS. They do reveal, however, the ways in which the context of crisis was having an impact on how forensic examination policy was being debated and implemented. Goldthorpe's suggestion that his colleagues should consider all addicts to be at high risk of HIV suggests an alarming and potentially coercive homogeneity of thought at work, whereby alcoholics or non-IV drug users may have been subjected to unnecessarily invasive questions, examinations or procedures relating to HIV.

This is despite the article suggesting that forensic examiners may happen 'upon the realisation that a person belongs to a "high risk" group'. The word 'realisation' is significant here, as it suggests a lack of clinical testing to reach such a conclusion. A patient's risk of HIV might be identified based on taking a detailed medical and/or sexual history or drawn from knowledge of their medical (or, indeed, criminal) record. But prejudiced assumptions may also have led police surgeons to such a 'realisation'. This is particularly significant given the fraught relationship between the police and several groups who were at especially high risk of contracting HIV during this period. Goldthorpe's article came just two years after the Chief Constable of Greater Manchester Police, James Anderton, suggested that drug users, sex workers and gay men with HIV were 'swirling around in a human cesspit of their own making' (Thomas 1993, 25–26). That he did so at a police seminar on AIDS further underlines the cultures of prejudice and fear, rather than evidence-based practices, within some British police forces during this period. Goldthorpe's article did not share Anderton's explicit homophobia, far from it, but it does suggest that some police surgeons may have relied on assumption

[3] That this referred specifically to the police is clear from figures taken just a few years after Goldthorpe's article was published which showed IV drug use was responsible for just 5% of HIV/AIDS cases in the UK, whereas sex between men accounted for 70% (Thomas 1993, 23).

or prejudice when identifying whether their patient/prisoners were at risk of having HIV.

For police surgeons, there were other means of ascertaining the HIV status of one's patient/prisoner. Of course, one could simply ask them. Doctors routinely asked their patients about their medical history, and the duty of care to those in their custody required police custody officers to enquire after their charges' physical and mental health following Code C of the 1984 Police and Criminal Evidence Act (Rekrut-Lapa and Lapa 2014, 69). As the experience of John Campbell with which this chapter opened demonstrates, such conversations could and did involve a discussion of HIV status. But when confronted with patients who, unlike Campbell, were unwilling or resisted coercion to undergo an HIV test, there were occasionally routes to discovering their HIV status which police surgeons were uniquely able to exploit. Goldthorpe revealed to his readership of fellow forensic examiners that 'on occasions' he had 'found the hospital willing to divulge to another doctor such details', namely 'the HIV status of the prisoner'. Of course, this was only possible 'if these are known already', that is, if the 'prisoner' had already undergone an HIV test previously (Goldthorpe 1988, 67).

Goldthorpe's suggestion here is a striking example of the crisis of consent police surgeons were experiencing around the issue of HIV testing. Once again, a close reading of the language employed begins to reveal its potentially coercive potential. To *divulge* something is to reveal a piece of sensitive information. From the Latin *vulgare* (to make known), modern definitions of the word emphasise the secret nature of the fact being broadcast. In Goldthorpe's context, the secret in question was the HIV status of his patient/prisoner, and the mechanism to make it known was the exploitation of the medical fraternity, exploitation which was required because his patient/prisoners had refused to reveal their HIV status to him. Asking the hospital to reveal the HIV status of the person they were dealing with was, as pitched by Goldthorpe at least, a last resort. Not only did this seem to stretch the physicians' professional obligation to confidentiality (something not mentioned by Goldthorpe), it explicitly used the police surgeon's medical qualification as a means to override this imperative. In other words, the police surgeon's medical expertise was being used directly as a tool of the criminal legal system to ascertain confidential medical information.

However, Goldthorpe's is a useful article through which to read the crisis of consent precisely because the consent of the patient/prisoner was emphasised. Goldthorpe was explicit on this point, telling his readers that patients were under 'no obligation to consent' to HIV testing (Ibid, 68). This further emphasises the importance of sexual violence cases as the theatres in which police surgeons rehearsed their arguments about HIV testing, as explored above. Discussing sexual assault cases, Goldthorpe's emphasis was more clearly directed at victims of rape being dealt with by his genitourinary medical colleagues rather than the alleged rapists whose care and evidence he had been responsible for. The need for consent, then, was absolute for victims in medical care, but was less definitive for those in the care of police surgeons or prison doctors. John Campbell's was not a sexual assault case, but it nonetheless underscores the fact that patient/prisoners could not always rely on their right not to consent to medical testing. Recall that Campbell was initially reluctant to undergo an HIV test but, having already done so previously, was told that 'you *have* to have another test' (emphasis added).

Without further research in this area, such as oral history interviews with police surgeons and patient/prisoners, historians must rely on informed conjecture when suggesting how coercively HIV testing was administered in criminal legal settings. In doing so, it is important to note that, when discussing sexual assault cases, Goldthorpe did emphasise the importance of consent. 'Should semen be involved' in sexual assault cases he dealt with, Goldthorpe wrote that 'I try to obtain, by consent, HIV and hepatitis B tests from the suspect, and phone my colleagues dealing with the other party' (that is, the victim, whose genitourinary referral he most likely made). A suspect might be persuaded to consent 'when it is explained that all that is required is a small blood sample', but Goldthorpe noted that 'this must be viewed in the light of any subsequent court proceedings and possible sentence'. Put another way, the blood sample may not be a major medical procedure, but it could make all the difference if it proved that a defendant had transmitted HIV to a complainant. As discussed above, this became a vital point for genitourinary medics to consider when they engaged with victims of rape and sexual assault.

Goldthorpe's article demonstrates the ways in which the primacy of consent, which had previously held firm and which he himself seemed to emphasise, could waiver in the face of HIV/AIDS anxieties. As HIV/AIDS became more endemic throughout the UK, the right of patient/prisoners to consent to be tested for the virus was questioned as an absolute by police surgeons. To be sure, there were areas of medical work within and outside of criminal legal settings in which patients' consent was not required. After the powers of the Public Health (Control of Disease) Act 1984 was extended to HIV/AIDS cases in 1985, medics were able to detain HIV positive patients in hospitals against their wishes, a 'draconian' power which was only used once (Berridge 1996, 71). However, obtaining blood samples consensually remained best practice when testing for HIV. Indeed, Goldthorpe's article demonstrated the ethical dance which the crisis of consent forced several police surgeons to perform, as the worsening HIV/AIDS epidemic increased the tension police surgeons experienced between the medical and juridical demands of their work.

Goldthorpe's revelation that police surgeons were using their medical status to obtain their patient/prisoners' HIV status suggested a less liberal element to this approach. Certainly this was more revealing of the ways in which the epidemic was altering police surgeons' thinking about the confidentiality of their patient/prisoners' medical information. There may have been some instances in which patients simply did not know the results of their previous HIV test (as in Campbell's case), and police surgeons were able to obtain them. However, whilst this remains a point of conjecture, it is not unreasonable to argue that on other such 'occasions', police surgeons were overriding their patient/prisoners' explicit lack of consent to provide them with that information. Where HIV was an issue for those in custody, consent and confidentiality's primacy was being questioned in illiberal and potentially coercive carceral settings.

## 5 Conclusion

Despite a crisis of consent in the mid-1980s, consent was a consistent feature in police surgeons' thinking about the HIV test. That crisis reveals the impacts of the culture of panic and anxiety which the HIV/AIDS epidemic, and the government's 'wartime response' to it, engendered amongst some police surgeons. More broadly, however, the picture of continuity which this chapter has painted—one in which the consent of the patient was underscored—has demonstrated the ways in which police surgeons and other medics dealing with cases which were both medical and criminal, formed liberal responses to the epidemic. Cases of non-consensual sex were crucial to the establishment of liberal medical policies around testing. Examining the formulation of this policy further reveals that the limits of that liberal response were felt most acutely within the criminal legal system: it was in the genitourinary units, rather than the police surgeons' examining suites, where patients' consent to HIV testing appears to have been most absolute. Unsurprisingly, it was in the coercive environment of the prison or custody suite that medics' emphasis on consent to an HIV test was most likely to waiver. The consistency of that emphasis, however, may further historical understandings of the distance police surgeons sought to place between themselves as medics and their 'police work' during this period. That distance, though, did not remove police surgeons' potential to use their medical status to override the consent and confidentiality of patients in their care. Indeed, the cases discussed in this chapter contribute to the growing body of scholarship which understands carcerality as a key factor in the erosion of its inhabitants' right to consent.

**Acknowledgements** I would like to thank the audience at the 2023 European Association for the History of Medicine and Health conference in Oslo, Norway for their insightful questions, as well as Joanna Bourke and Rhian Keyse for their perceptive and helpful notes on earlier drafts of this chapter.

**Funding** This work was supported by the Wellcome Trust (grant ID 205378/Z/16/Z), as part of the Sexual Harms and Medical Encounters project. The authors declare no competing interests.

## References

### Primary Sources

Book Review: Herpes, AIDS and Other Sexually Transmitted Diseases. Derek Llewellyn-Jones. 1985. *The Police Surgeon* 28: 79–80.

Minutes of the 34th Annual General Meeting held at the Golden Valley Hotel, Cheltenham on 15th May 1985'. 1986. *The Police Surgeon Supplement* 20: 16–17.

Recording HIV Status on Police Computers. 1992. *British Medical Journal* 304: 1243.

Burges, H., and J. E. Hilton, eds. 1978. *The New Police Surgeon: A Practical Guide to Clinical Forensic Medicine*. London: Hutchinson Benham.

Cancer Research Campaign Working Party in Breast Conservation. 1983. Informed Consent: Ethical, Legal, and Medical Implications for Doctors and Patients Who Participate in Randomised Clinical Trials. *British Medical Journal (Clinical Research Edition)* 286: 1117–1121. https://doi.org/10/1136/bmj.286.6371.1117

Doll, Richard. 1987. A Proposal for Drug Prevalence Studies of AIDS. *British Medical Journal (Clinical Research Edition)* 294: 244. https://doi.org/10.1136.bmj.294.6566.244

Foster, Ilene, and John G. Bartlett. 1989. Rape and Subsequent Seroconversion to HIV. *British Medical Journal* 299: 1282.

Gillon, Raanan. 1987. Testing for HIV Without Permission. *British Medical Journal (Clinical Research Edition)* 294: 821–823. https://doi.org/10.1136/bmj.294.6575.821.

Goldthorpe, S. B. 1988. AIDS and the Police Surgeon. *The Police Surgeon* 33: 64–69.

Hillman, Richard, Nigel O'Mara, and David Tomlinson. 1991. Adult Male Victims of Sexual Assault: An Underdiagnosed Condition. *International Journal of STD & AIDS* 2: 22–24.

Hilton, J. E. 1986. AIDS and the Police. *The Police Surgeon* 30: 120–123.

John Campbell interviewed by Wendy Rickard 30th September 1996, British Library Sound Archive: C743/09, tape 4 (F5463), side A.

Mason, J. K. 1992. Recording HIV Status on Police Computers. *British Medical Journal* 304: 995–996.

Murphy, S. V., J. R. W. Harris. Kitchen, and S. M. Forster. 1989. Rape and Subsequent Seroconversion to HIV. *British Medical Journal* 299: 718.

Roberts, Raine. 1986. STD—When Should the First Check Be Made? *The Police Surgeon Supplement* 21: 31.

Roberts, Raine. 1987. St Mary's Centre. *The Police Surgeon Supplement* 22: 46–47.

Tobias, J. S. and R. L. Souhami. 1993. Fully Informed Consent Can Be Needlessly Cruel. *British Medical Journal* 307: 1199–1201.https://doi.org/10/1136/bmj.307.6913.1199.

## Secondary Sources

Berridge, Virginia. 1996. *AIDS in the UK: The Making of Policy, 1981–1994.* Oxford: Oxford University Press.

Bourke, Joanna. 2007. *Rape: A History from 1860 to the Present*. London: Virago.

Bourke, Joanna. 2018. Police Surgeons and Victims of Rape: Cultures of Harm and Care. *Social History of Medicine* 31 (4): 711–731.

Cook, Matt. 2017a. AIDS, Mass Observation, and the Fate of the Permissive Turn. *Journal of the History of Sexuality* 26: 239–272.

Cook, Matt. 2017b. "Archives of Feeling": The AIDS Crisis in Britain 1987. *History Workshop Journal* 83: 51–78.

Cox, Pamela. 2007. Compulsion, Voluntarism, and Venereal Disease: Governing Sexual Health in England after the Contagious Diseases Acts. *Journal of British Studies* 46: 91–115.

Day, Emma. 2023. *In Her Hands: Women's Fight against AIDS in the United States*. Berkley, CA: University of California Press.

Dirven, Pauline. 2024. Detached from Sympathy, Unconscious of Trauma: The Impact of the Forensic Virtues of Impartiality and Detachment on Rape Examinations in Britain 1924–1978. *Social History of Medicine* 37: 494–515. https://doi.org/10.1093/shm/hkad097.

Dodds, Catherine, Adam Bourne, and Matthew Weait. 2009. Responses to Criminal Prosecutions for HIV Transmission Among Gay Men with HIV in England and Wales. *Reproductive Health Matters* 17: 135–145.

Elizabeth, Hannah J. 2022. Recovering Mothers' Experiences of HIV/AIDS Health Activism in Edinburgh, 1983–2000. In *Histories of HIV/AIDS in Western Europe: New and Regional Perspectives*, ed. Janet Weston and Hannah J. Elizabeth, 164–191. Manchester: Manchester University Press.

Laite, Julia. 2012. *Common Prostitutes and Ordinary Citizens: Commercial Sex in London, 1885–1960*. Basingstoke: Palgrave Macmillan.

Lee, Sandra S-J., Mildred J. Cho, Stephanie A. Kraft, Nina Varsava, Katie Gillespie, Kelly E. Ormond, Benjamin S. Wilfond, and David Magnus. 2019. "I Don't Want to be Henrietta Lacks": Diverse Patient Perspectives on Donating Biospecimens for Precision Medicine Research. *Genetics in Medicine* 21: 107–113.

Levin, Benjamin. 2023. After The Criminal Justice System. *Washington Law Review* 98 (3): 899–946.

Reed, Jeremy. 2013. *The Dilly: A History of the Piccadilly Rent Boy Scene*. London: Peter Owns.

Rekrut-Lapa, Tatyana, and Alexander Lapa. 2014. Health Needs of Detainees in Police Custody in England and Wales. Literature Review. *Journal of Forensic and Legal Medicine* 27: 69–75.

Rusterholz, Caroline and Laura Kelly. 2025. Depo-Provera, Class, Race, and the Domiciliary Family Planning Services in Glasgow and Haringey, 1970–1983. *Historical Journal* 68, 216–238.

Severs, George J. 2024a. *Radical Acts: HIV/AIDS Activism in Late-Twentieth Century England*. London: Bloomsbury Academic.

Severs, George J. 2024b. Male Rape: Survivors, Support and the Law in Late Twentieth-Century England and Wales. *History Workshop Journal* 97: 196–220.

Slagstad, Ketil and Anne Kveim Lie. 2022. Selling Sex in the Age of HIV/AIDS: Activism, Politics, and Medicine in Norway, 1983–90. In *Histories of HIV/AIDS in Western Europe: New and Regional Perspectives*, ed. Janet Weston and Hannah J. Elizabeth, 27–58. Manchester: Manchester University Press.

Thomas, Philip A. 1993. The Nuclear Family, Ideology and AIDS in the Thatcher Years. *Feminist Legal Studies* 1: 23–44.

Thomlinson, Natalie. 2016. *Race, Ethnicity and the Women's Movement in England, 1968–1993*. Basingstoke: Palgrave Macmillan.

Ware, Cheryl. 2019. *HIV Survivors in Sydney: Memories of the Epidemic*. Cham: Palgrave Macmillan.

Weston, Janet. 2019. Sites of Sickness, Sites of Rights? HIV/AIDS and the Limits of Human Rights in British Prisons'. *Cultural and Social History* 16 (2): 225–240.

Weston, Janet. 2022. Responding to HIV/AIDS in European Prisons, 1980s–2000s. In *Histories of HIV/AIDS in Western Europe: New and Regional Perspectives*, ed. Janet Weston and Hannah J. Elizabeth, 82–108. Manchester: Manchester University Press.

## Online Sources

Laurie, Graeme. 2017, February 6. Obituary: Professor Ken Mason, Medical Jurisprudence Pioneer. *The Scotsman*. https://www.scotsman.com/news/obituary-professor-ken-mason-medical-jurisprudence-pioneer-1456658. Accessed on 12 September 2023.

# Index






R. E. Keyse et al. (eds.), *Sexual Violence in Medicine and Psychiatry*, Genders and Sexualities in History, https://doi.org/10.1007/978-3-032-10800-5

## H



## I



## J



## K


Kaladelfos, Andy, 6, 64, 66–69, 79


## L



## M

The manufacturer's authorised representative in the EU is Springer Nature Customer Service Centre GmbH, Europaplatz 3, 69115 Heidelberg, Germany. If you have any concerns regarding our products, please contact ProductSafety@springernature.com

Printed and bound by CPI Group (UK) Ltd, Croydon, CR0 4YY

21/09/2026

02220011-0006